mHealth in Practice

Mobile technology for health promotion in the developing world

Edited by
Jonathan Donner
and
Patricia Mechael

BLOOMSBURY
LONDON • NEW DELHI • NEW YORK • SYDNEY

Bloomsbury Academic
An imprint of Bloomsbury Publishing Plc

50 Bedford Square
London
WC1B 3DP
UK

175 Fifth Avenue
New York
NY 10010
USA

www.bloomsbury.com

First published 2013

CIP records for this book are available from the British Library and the Library of Congress

ISBN: PB: 978-1-78093-229-3

Printed and bound in Great Britain by MPG Books Group, Bodmin, Cornwall.

Acknowledgments

As the co-editors of this volume, Patricia Mechael and Jonathan Donner would like to extend our appreciation to the commitment of our respective institutional homes, the Earth Institute at Columbia University and Microsoft Research, for encouraging us in this endeavor. A debt of gratitude is owed most especially to the project management leadership of Nadi Kaonga, whose day-to-day management of the work of the authors and editors alike kept us all on track and focused. This book would not have been possible without the support, enthusiasm, and participation of each of the contributing authors – most of which are practitioners who willingly carved out the time and mental space for research, writing, and reflection. We gratefully appreciate Bloomsbury Academic for publishing this volume and especially for the thoughtful guidance of Frances Pinter and James Powell.

We would also like to thank the GSMA and most especially Chris Locke and his colleagues, Philippa Zamora, Hayley Minett, Richard Cockle, and Gavin Krugel, for their financial and consultative contribution that made it possible for the authors represented in this book to meet in the United Kingdom to collectively advance their chapters and reflect on the lessons they have gleaned from implementing a broad range of mHealth for behavior change initiatives. Similarly, we thank colleagues at Royal Holloway and ICTD2010, namely Tim Unwin, Dorothea Kleine, Caitlin Bentley, and Sandie Venables; and the London School of Hygiene and Tropical Medicine, namely Andy Haines and Caroline Free as well as Phil Edwards, Maria Perez, and Robert Lovesey, for providing a forum for public and private dialogue. Thank you to Jaclyn Carlsen and Erica Kochi for helping us to capture people's thoughts during the ICTD2010 mHealthy Behaviors Workshop and Grass Roots Group's Julie Yorke, Sue Shearman, Debbie King, Francesca Sands, Nicola Hayhoe, and Jane Carvalho for helping everyone to find their way to and from the United Kingdom despite the snowy weather.

At Microsoft Research, we would like to express our appreciation for the efforts and support of Ed Cutrell, Kentaro Toyama, Bill Thies, P. Anandan, Kristin Tolle, Vidya Natampally, Ashwani Sharma, Sarah Nightingale, Mari Ann Lindqvist, Chris Gould-Sandhu, and Sachin Agarwal. At the Earth Institute, we are grateful to Jeffrey Sachs, Sonia Sachs, Joanna Rubinstein, Vijay Modi, Andrew Kanter, Matt Berg, and Nadi Kaonga. Of our professional colleagues, we want to especially thank Claire O'Neill, June Flora, James Katz, BJ Fogg, Alison Bloch, Deb Levine, and Josh Ruxin.

Patty would like to thank her parents, Mona and Nagi Mechael, for showing her that every journey begins with a single step; her sisters Sandy and Anne for keeping her honest; and Merrick Schaefer for his inspiration and our mBaby-Gabriel Sabry who has benefited greatly from mobile messaging before and since his birth. Jonathan would like to thank his family, particularly Caitlin and Calliope, Karen and Richard, Ann and Chris, for their patience and support over the long nights, long trips, and long hauls that comprise a research career.

It is our sincere hope that this volume finds itself into the hands of students, practitioners, health policymakers, researchers, and all those with an interest in leveraging the power of mobile to improve health and well-being and provides thoughtful insights that inform the shaping of the next generation of mHealth for behavior change deployments.

Contents

List of Tables and Figures

Tables

Figures

Notes on Contributors

Hajo van Beijma is the partnership director of the Text to Change Foundation (TTC). In 2007 Hajo co-founded TTC with two colleagues and started with an office in Uganda and the Netherlands. TTC has since then executed more than twenty successful mHealth programs targeting 3,000,000 mobile phone users with health sensitization messages in Uganda, Kenya, Tanzania, and Namibia and is expanding to fifteen countries in Africa and South America. Hajo is the co-author of several publications on mHealth.

Peter Benjamin is the managing director of Cell-Life. For twenty years he has worked with information and communications technology for social change, now focusing on 'mHealth'. Dr Benjamin moved to South Africa (SA) from the United Kingdom in 1994. He has a first degree in physics, a Master's in IT and his PhD examined universal access to ICTs through telecenters. He is married to Marion Stevens, and has two wonderful boys (Joel and Xanny). Peter is on the executive of the SA Telemedicine Association, is the treasurer of the People's Health Movement of SA, is a member of the SA ICT4Health stakeholder forum, and is a member of the Treatment Action Campaign.

Heather Cole-Lewis earned her PhD Candidate in Chronic Disease Epidemiology from Yale School of Public Health and her Master of Public Health in Behavioral Science and Health Education from Emory University Rollins School of Public Health. Heather's interests include improving the design, research, and evaluation of information communication technology health interventions. She has published in several peer-reviewed journals, including Epidemiologic Reviews, American Journal of Public Health, and International Journal for Quality in Health Care.

Jonathan Donner is a researcher in the Technology for Emerging Markets Group (TEM) at Microsoft Research, India. With research focused on the economic and social implications of the spread of mobile telephony in the developing world, his projects at TEM include microenterprise/MSE development, mobile banking, mobile health and well-being, and 'first time/mobile-only' internet use. His PhD is from Stanford University in Communication Research. He is the author, with Richard Ling, of Mobile Communication (Polity, 2009). His research also appears in the Journal of Computer-Mediated Communication, the Information Society, the Journal of Information Technologies and International Development, the Journal of International Development, and Innovations: Technology, Governance, Globalization.

Dr Caroline Free is a researcher in the Clinical Trials Unit at the London School of Hygiene and Tropical Medicine and a general practitioner. Her research is in the development and evaluation of health communication interventions with a current focus on using mobile technologies to deliver interventions to support people in adopting healthy behaviors or self-manage aspects of disease. She was the principal investigator for the txt2stop trial which was published in the Lancet. This trial showed that text messaging support doubles biochemically verified quitting at six months. She has also published in the BMJ, WHO bulletin, and other health journals.

Jose Gomez-Marquez leads the Little Devices lab at the Massachusetts Institute of Technology and is the co-founder of LDTC+Labs LLC. The Little Devices group explores the design, invention, and policy spaces for DIY health technologies around the world. The research portfolio includes Adhere.IO, a patient-centric platform for remote medication adherence and the MEDIKit, a series of design building blocks that empower doctors and nurses in developing countries to invent their medical technologies. His work has appeared in the IEEE Spectrum, Make Magazine, Wired, and Technology Review.

Bas Hoefman is the founder and director of Text to Change (TTC). Back in 2006, while working as a banker, he was inspired by the growth of mobile technology in Africa from which he discovered the potential of using mobile technology for health education. He co-founded Text to Change with two colleagues with whom he implemented the first mHealth project in 2008. Since then, Bas has been heading the TTC Africa office from Kampala, Uganda. TTC has led the way in using interactive text messaging for health in Africa and has so far implemented over twenty successful mHealth programs.

Nadi Nina Kaonga is a graduate of Columbia University, where she obtained a Bachelors of Arts in neuroscience and behavior. She has a Masters in Health Science degree from the Department of International Health's Global Disease Epidemiology and Control Program at the Johns Hopkins University Bloomberg School of Public Health. Nadi has worked with researchers at the Earth Institute (EI) since 2009. Her roles at EI have evolved from serving as a 'mIntern' (or mobile health (mHealth) intern) to mHealth Program Coordinator to Research and

Evaluation Coordinator. Nadi has spent time in her home country of Malawi, working on projects including the prevention of mother-to-child transmission of HIV/AIDS and, separately, mHealth initiatives. Most recently, she conducted an assessment of the mobile phone closed user group in the Millennium Villages Project site of Bonsaaso, Ghana, while continuing to support and coordinate the OASIS Research Project activities and the Ghana Telemedicine Project.

Ada Kwan is a researcher in the Center of Evaluation Research and Surveys at the Mexican National Institute of Public Health, where she has been involved in economic, impact, and efficiency evaluations primarily for improving HIV/AIDS service delivery and financial incentive schemes in countries in Africa and Latin America. Her experience and interests also include qualitative research and analysis on how mobile phones can be utilized to improve particularly maternal and child health care services and HIV/AIDS and tuberculosis disease management. She is a co-author on the policy white paper entitled 'Barriers and gaps affecting mHealth in low- and middle-income countries' by Mechael, Batavia, Kaonga, Searle, Kwan, Fu, and Ossman (2010).

Ilta Lange is professor and director of the WHO/PAHO Collaborating Center for Primary Health Care at the School of Nursing at the Pontificia Universidad Católica de Chile. With financial support from the National Science Fund (FONDEF D04i1171), she implemented the Laboratory for Remote Health Care (LRHC) at the School of Nursing in 2005. An interdisciplinary healthcare team of nurses, a psychologist, a physician, a nutritionist, and an engineer have been working together since its creation, to design and implement tele self-management support models for patients with Type 2 diabetes. Over the years, Professor Lange and her colleagues have received additional funding support for their research projects and feasibility studies from the National Science Fund/FONIS projects, the Chilean Ministry of Health, local health services, and the Inter American Development Bank.

Patricia Mechael is the Executive Director of the mHealth Alliance, which is hosted by the United Nations Foundation, and faculty at the School of International and Public Affairs and Earth Institute, Columbia University. Prior to joining the mHealth Alliance, she was Director of Strategic Application of Mobile Technology for Public Health and Development at the Center for Global Health and Economic Development at the Earth Institute. Since 1996, she has been actively involved in the field of international health with field experience of over thirty countries primarily in Africa, the Middle East, and Asia. For over ten years, Dr Mechael has published and spoken extensively on the strategic role of mobile telephony and relevant software applications within an ecosystem of eHealth, public health, and telecommunications actors in low- and middle-income countries as well as the increasing need to engage women and girls more effectively in designing and implementing the solutions aimed at improving their health and quality of life. She has a Master's in international health from the Johns Hopkins School of Public Health and Hygiene (1998) and a PhD in public health and policy from the London School of Hygiene and Tropical Medicine (2006), where she specifically examined the role of mobile phones in relation to health in Egypt.

Permanand Mohan is a senior lecturer in computer science in the Department of Computing and Information Technology at the University of the West Indies, St Augustine Campus in Trinidad and Tobago. Dr Mohan was the principal investigator of a mobile health remote monitoring project for patients suffering from diabetes and cardiovascular disease in the Caribbean. The project was funded by Microsoft Research as part of its 'Cellular Phone as a Platform for Healthcare' RFP. He presently supervises several postgraduate students in the areas of mobile health, mobile learning, e-learning, and games for learning/health. His research has appeared in a number of conference proceedings, book chapters, and in journals such as the e-Minds Journal of Human Computer Interaction, Computational Intelligence, and the International Journal of Mobile Learning and Organization.

Jessica Osborn has spent five years working on mobile innovation in Uganda, Ghana, and Mali. In Uganda, she worked with the Grameen Foundation and partners MTN and Google to create some of the apps in the Google SMS suite and test out sustainable business models for rural internet access. She spent almost three years with the Grameen Foundation in Ghana, managing a project to create mobile services to improve maternal and child health, in partnership with the Ghana Health Service. Jess currently works on Mobile Financial Services with Tigo in Ghana. Prior to joining the world of mobile, Jess worked with Cisco Systems in London and Dubai on their corporate responsibility team. Jess graduated in politics, economics, and sociology from Durham University in England.

Hilmi Quraishi is a co-founder of ZMQ Software, and an Ashoka fellow. He is the prime architect of 'Freedom HIV/AIDS', a mobile phone games initiative to create awareness on HIV/AIDS. ZMQ has created over eighty social games and implemented twelve targeted mobile phone interventions on healthcare in India and Africa. Under the 'Mobile for All' initiative, Hilmi is advocating for 'Universal Right to Connectivity' as a 'Right to Life' to provide free primary healthcare services to underprivileged and rural communities in India.

Subhi Quraishi is the CEO of ZMQ Software, an India-based social enterprise. Subhi is a 'Technology for Development' expert who specializes in developing mobile technology solutions in low-resource settings. Subhi has graduated from open-ended information delivery on mobile phones to targeted interventions such as disease management, patient tracking, rural financial services, and life-line services, which has been christened as OHM@BoP – 'Organized Human Networks @ Bottom of the Pyramid'. He is also leading two new initiatives under ZMQ called "EmpowerShe" - unveiling women using mobile technology, and "Qaff Games" - multi-platform social games initiative.

Divya Ramachandran completed her PhD at the University of California, Berkeley, where she researched the use of mobile phone videos to assist community health workers in rural India. She has conducted research in the areas of mobile health and persuasive technologies and published her work in the proceedings of conferences such as Human Factors in Computing, Persuasive, and Information and Communications Technologies and Development. She currently works as a user experience designer at Marketo, Inc.

Salys Sultan is a PhD candidate and assistant lecturer in the Department of Computing and Information Technology at the University of the West Indies, St Augustine Campus. Her PhD thesis surrounds the use of mobile technologies for patient self-care management. Her research interests include modeling and design of mobile applications, computer-supported ubiquitous learning, and advanced technology in education. She has worked on two mobile health initiatives; MediNet: A Mobile Healthcare Management System for the Caribbean Region, and Mobile DSMS: A Peer-Facilitated Diabetes Self-Management Support System. For more information about her research interests and publications, please visit http://www.salys.org.

1 mHealthy Behaviors

Engaging researchers and practitioners in a facilitated dialogue on mobile-mediated health behavior change

Patricia Mechael, mHealth Alliance at the UN Foundation and Earth Institute at Columbia University
Jonathan Donner, Microsoft Research

Introduction

From diagnostics to disease surveillance to telemedicine, there is an explosion of interest regarding the application of mobile communication technologies to support health initiatives. One topic garnering particular enthusiasm is the use of mobile telephones to support and promote healthy behaviors and to prevent unhealthy behaviors. These behavioral support and change initiatives are particularly challenging (and promising) when applied to resource-constrained settings where other forms of outreach and messaging are not cost-effective, and where few other channels for customized outreach (digital or otherwise) are available. In the first decade of the twenty-first century, billions of people have purchased the first telephone of their lives – clearly there are opportunities to leverage these new connections for public health.

As mobile phone-based health promotion activities and campaigns increase in scale and momentum, understanding the pathways to behavior change and the role of mobile technology is essential. This is not simply an abstract theoretical exercise, but rather a matter of immediate practical concern as programs need to be developed, protocols approved, and change pursued. Yet it seems that there are few opportunities for exchange of information and proven practice between practitioners and researchers. At the moment, there is limited knowledge among practitioners on best practices and how best to optimize or evaluate the role of mobile-mediated interactions as they relate to health behavior change.

To support this need, the Technology for Emerging Markets Group (TEM) at Microsoft Research India and the Center for Global Health and Development (CGHED) at the Earth Institute at Columbia University hosted a workshop and roundtable in London, from 16 to 17 December 2010, called mHealthy Behaviors: using mobile phones to support and promote healthy behaviors in the developing world. Travel support was provided by MSR India and a generous grant from the GSMA Development Fund, with extensive additional technical support provided by CGHED. The first day of the event was an open session held in conjunction with the 4th International Conference on Information and Communication Technologies and Development (ICTD2010) conference at Royal Holloway Campus of the University of London[1]. The second day was a closed-door roundtable hosted by London School of Hygiene and Tropical Medicine. Representing mobile-mediated behavioral change and support projects in Latin America, Africa, Europe, and South Asia, the contributors included mHealth practitioners from NGOs and the private sector, as well as researcher/practitioners from leading academic institutions.

The first goal of the sessions was to give practitioners an opportunity to make their implicit change models regarding the use of mobile technologies for behavior change and health promotion explicit, and to identify best practices for implementation as well as research priorities for the future. The second goal was to begin to craft the chapters in this volume.

The conversations in the United Kingdom and the accompanying background papers provided the basis for the original chapters on mobile-enabled behavioral change included in this volume. For some of our authors, this was a rare opportunity to document their experiences for their colleagues in the mHealth field, to explore behavior change and communication models, and to position their experiences within the context of other programs and research of relevance to their areas of practice. In other cases, behavioral researchers and epidemiologists working in the areas of mHealth and behavior change were engaged to share their own learning on what is working or not when it comes to evaluating the impact of such programs.

The domain of mediated behavior change is, of course, not new. There is a rich tradition of research and practice of mass media behavior change campaigns (Rice and Atkin, 2001; Hornick, 2002; Siegel and Lotenberg, 2004). Yet interactive channels such as computers and mobile phones bring new issues to the fore and may not be adequately addressed by established social marketing paradigms (Lefebvre and Flora, 1988). Thus, the closest volumes available now are from the internet space (Rice and Katz, 2001) and from the mobile field (Fogg and Eckles, 2007; Fogg and Adler, 2009). The latter is an excellent, accessible volume by leaders in the field. However – similar to much of the literature available on mHealth – Fogg and Alder do not focus on developing countries, nor do they directly interrogate what works and what does not work with an eye toward best practices Mechael, Batavia, Kaonga, Searle, Kwan, Fu, and Ossman (2010). Chapter two by Kwan, Mechael, and Kaonga in this volume aims to bridge this gap in the literature and pulls from existing sources as well as the work of contributing authors and other practitioners using mobile to promote healthier behaviors.

The mHealthy behaviors sessions

This work began in direct response to the ample programming, increasing hype, and recognizable gap within the mHealth literature of what works and how it works when it comes to programs that aim to leverage mobile technology to engage individuals in stopping an unhealthy behavior or taking up an activity that would preserve their well-being and prevent the onset of illness and disease. With rapid increases in funding for such programs, particularly in low and middle income countries – where the health disparities are greatest – the need to unlock the secrets to the pathways to change became increasingly apparent. To start, we began by combing the literature and mHealth community for projects and research that could tell the mobile-mediated behavior change story from multiple angles – particularly from the perspective of those of practitioners implementing such programs and researchers evaluating their impact. We also wanted to address the 'do-know' gap in mHealth, whereby the majority of programs are being implemented in low and middle income countries with the majority of research and evaluation coming from high-income settings (Mechael and Searle, 2010). We also wanted to ensure geographic representation to compare and contrast the maturity of mHealth, cultural, language, and socio-economic considerations. It was through these lenses that authors and their respective projects and research were selected and invited to participate in what would become a nine-month long reflective exercise, which ultimately led to the full development of the chapters included in this book.

The projects and authors involved in this effort are as follows:

Table 1.1 Authors and subjects

Author(s)	Organization	Chapter Description
Caroline Free	London School of Hygiene and Tropical Medicine	Outlines the methodology and processes used to develop the txt2stop intervention in the UK
Divya Ramachandran	University of California, Berkeley	Provides the author's personal experience and work on addressing rural maternal health issues using mobile persuasive messages in India
Hajo van Beijma and Bas Hoefman	Text to Change	Highlights positive feedback and challenges of Text to Change's early pilot and scale-up efforts of SMS campaigns in Uganda

Continued

Table 1.1 Continued

Author(s)	Organization	Chapter Description
Heather Cole-Lewis	Yale School of Public Health	Details the author's reasons for and experience in conducting a systematic review of literature on the use of text messaging as a tool for behavior change and disease management in a global context
Ilta Lange	Catholic University of Chile	Reflection on lessons learned from a tele-care initiative on self-management support of patients with Type 2 diabetes in Chile
Jessica Osborn	Grameen App Lab	Early lessons learned from one of the first fully implemented projects in mHealth – Mobile Technology for Community Health (MoTECH) in Ghana
Jose Gomez-Marquez	Massachusetts Institute of Technology	Underscores challenges and evolution of an approach to TB treatment adherence
Peter Benjamin	Cell-Life	Personal account of initiating and expanding HIV communications in the ICT field in South Africa
Salys Sultan and Permanand Mohan	University of the West Indies	Personal account from software developers in mHealth, working on the MediNet Project in the Caribbean
Subhi Quraishi and Hilmi Quraishi	ZMQ Software	Details experiences in developing mobile phone games for health communication, with a focus on HIV/AIDS, in India

While we specifically targeted this effort to focus on the use of mobile technologies for behavior change in developing countries, we included the work of Free at the London School of Hygiene and Tropical Medicine as the use of text messaging is increasingly being incorporated in smoking cessation campaigns throughout the world. The rigorous intervention design and research provides an excellent case study of what mHealth for behavior change initiatives ought to aspire toward as many now seek to transition from pilots to scale.

To begin this process, we invited each author to develop an abstract and/or short outline that addressed the following (deceptively simple) question: what is it that you intended to do, and why/how did you believe it would work? Related questions for authors included:

- Did/does your project have a specific model of behavior change? If so, how did you match your design to this model?
- Where did you go for guidance? What literature or other projects were influential? Is your model unique to 'mobile' behavior change or does it draw on/inform broader behavior change models?
- Conversely, how did the project execution inform your model? How did it evolve over time? Did you make any mid-course adjustments? Would you use the model again?
- How was your change model reflected in your evaluation plans?
- What methods did you use to assess the success of your program? To what extent were you able to measure changes in behavior?
- What recommendations might you make to program implementers and evaluators based on your experience?

The back-to-back workshop and roundtable included a discussion on the need for practitioners to engage both with formal behavior change theory and with the more iterative, natural pursuit of technological and organizational best practices, a gap that many in the medical (Lomas, 2007), education Amabile, Patterson, Mueller, Wojcik, Odomirok, Marsh, and Kramer (2001), and management (Amabile, Patterson, Mueller *et al.*, 2001) communities have argued can be hard to bridge. It involved a 'reflective spirit' of interactive discussion (Schön, 1983; Argyris, Putnam and Smith, 1985) with elements of action research, a focus on guided discussion, open exchange, and reflection. Pre-work included reading excerpts of the Reflective Practitioner (Schön, 1983), and made references to the theatrical practice of 'breaking frame' (for example, Kantor and Hoffman, 1966) and to Failfare[2], the set of ICT4D meetings in which failed projects are scrutinized, celebrated, and used as the basis for rapid learning. Returning to that deceptively simple question, part one (what is it you intended to do?) promised to bring us along well-trod paths in workshop settings, while part two (why did you believe it would work?) offered more opportunities for reflection, and more explicit links to change models (Frumkin, 2006). Many of the change models utilized by the contributing authors were done without prior or formal articulation; only a few had proactively researched and applied explicit strategies for behavioral change.

The half-day workshop was open to attendees at ICTD2010, hosted at the Royal Holloway campus of the University of London. Eleven invited panelists from around the world shared their experiences in a format that actively engaged the audience, including other mHealth practitioners and researchers, in the discussions. The sessions followed a 'fish-bowl' design; audience participants moved in and out of the discussion by taking a seat among the panelists. This session enabled us to gain a sense of the interest levels in the broader ICTD community, as well as to identify questions that we ought to consider ensuring that we tackle within this volume. Notes from this session are available on the public website for this reflective writing collaboration[3].

The second session was a full-day, closed-door roundtable at the London School of Hygiene and Tropical Medicine (also a part of the University of London). In preparation of the closed session, we provided targeted feedback to each of the authors to expand their abstracts to 3,500 – 6,000 word documents. The bulk of the roundtable was spent walking through change models and the application of theoretical frameworks to the various projects and research and discussing the paper drafts from participants. Practitioners and researchers in the mHealth domain were asked to approach their practice from a variety of perspectives, mixing formal or implicit theory (of behavior change, in this case), with intuition and adjustment on the fly. Numerous commentators have defined such approaches as 'change models'.

mHealthy behavioral themes

This introductory chapter highlights many of the themes that emerged throughout the process of developing this edited volume and draws heavily on the public and private dialogue of the authors along with other mHealth and mobile communication practitioners. The following chapter provides the context out of which the programs described in this book grew, including an overview of the state of the mHealth and mHealth for behavior change fields. For the practitioner chapter contributions, each of the author experiences fell into one or more of the following themes:

- Designing for individuals is different from designing for caregivers.
- Technology-supported behavior change and support requires a multidisciplinary team.
- Calibrate for the low end vs. the high end of the technical landscape.

- Organizations matter. Ensure buy-in and openness.
- Start with scale in mind. Decide if failure is an option.
- Local context matters.
- Link theory to practice via behavior change models.
- The elusive art of measuring change.

Designing for patients is different from designing for caregivers

Some of the authors and workshop participants highlighted the differences between deploying mHealth solutions for caregivers and for individuals. The descriptions of ALTAS in Chile (by Lange) and MOTECH in Ghana (by Osborn) describe how the single systems had both a caregiver and a patient component, developed somewhat simultaneously. Cole-Lewis's paper correctly captures the essence of this distinction – 'even when the goal in any case may be behavioral change or support, we cannot skip from use of technology to measuring health outcomes, without understanding the mechanism of change by which we expect the health outcomes to improve'. Interventions focused on patients are different from interventions focused on providers, and demand different designs and evaluation methods.

For designers perhaps more familiar with working in organizational settings with people relatively more like them – nurses, doctors, managers – the shift to designing for end-users may require even more engagement and listening. Discussion at the workshops suggested that focus groups and follow ups could uncover mismatches between the assumptions of designers and the end-users (Heeks, 2002), such as the stigmas around reminders vs. the opportunity to develop self-esteem though positive messages, as discovered by many of the contributing authors. As Gomez-Marquez explained, securing user involvement (for example, participatory design processes (Sjöberg and Timpka, 1998)) right from the beginning was critical. By engaging users as designers, face-to-face beside the designer not in front of them during interviews (or worse, kept at a distance via mediated surveys and remote consultations), more optimal directions were discovered, including the opportunity to use cellphone minutes (airtime) as a reward and incentive.

Technology-supported behavior change and support requires a multidisciplinary team

Sultan and Mohan, Gomez-Marquez, Benjamin, and Cole-Lewis underscore how the development and deployment of a mobile-mediated behavior change initiative is, like most ICT initiatives in healthcare, a multidisciplinary undertaking

(Bakker, 2002). Sultan and Mohan were computer scientists with an inkling of a great idea, but without the help of a medical doctor, their initiative to craft a system to support diabetes care and treatment would not go far. Similarly, Benjamin described how important it was for their team of electrical engineers to work with a medical doctor – not as much for insights into end-users. In their case, the value was to allow for insights into how to work effectively within the national healthcare system and its associated bureaucracies. For the Adhere.IO project, Gomez-Marquez described the formation of a multidisciplinary team that combined 'chemistry, mechanical engineering, policy, economics, and clinical experience. Beyond creating diversity in the group, we forced cross-functional tasks to avoid attacking the problem conventionally. In fact we did not have an IT person at the inception of the project.'

In the discussion of her systematic literature review, Cole-Lewis also broached the multidisciplinary issue, from a different angle. Not only are teams multidisciplinary, but so must be metrics and meta-analyses. Cole-Lewis could not count on a standardized set of metrics from the studies she assessed; they came from different disciplines, and had different approaches to assessment and evaluation.

Calibrate for the low end versus the high end of the technical landscape

Some people have smartphones. Some people have basic phones, capable of only voice calls and text messaging. However, a lot of people have something in-between – one of hundreds of different configurations of 'feature phones' capable of running some software, snapping a picture, accessing a simple web page, or playing back a video. A challenge for many mHealth projects in resource constrained settings is that the ratios of smartphones: feature phones: basic phones are shifting. As Benjamin describes in detail, practitioners must elect whether to proceed with a lowest common denominator approach (voice calls, IVR, SMS, USSD), or to build and deploy against higher expectations of users' handsets and network capabilities, using data, images, software, video, etc. As with the case in other development domains, like livelihoods and agricultural information systems (Donner, 2009), there is no correct answer; only a caution that the set of options must be evaluated before a choice is made. What made sense for Text-to-Change (SMS messages to potentially every user in a geographic area) was not the same as what made sense for Ramachandran (prenatal care videos loaded on the handsets of healthcare workers, who then shared them by sitting alongside pregnant women and mothers).

Osborn's chapter offered a detailed description of the trade-offs Grameen made in Ghana when selecting handsets for the nursing component of a project leveraging mobile phones to facilitate reporting from clinics for maternal and child health. They elected to provide dedicated feature phones to nurses in their program, while end-users in the midwives program accessed their parts of the system using IVR. For the demands of the nurse's system SMS would have been expensive (on a per message basis), insecure, and hard to customize. Despite unease with providing dedicated handsets to nurses, the flexibility of the Java environment on the feature phones made the choice worthwhile.

But feature phones are not just for caregivers and dedicated users; Quraishi and Quraishi's chapter on mobile games in India suggests that scale can be achieved with initiatives targeting feature phone end-users, as well. They describe a suite of mobile games, calibrated to run on popular feature phone handset models and hosted by Reliance (a major network in India). Once the games became available on other networks, over 40 million users had potential access; ZMQ logged over ten million game sessions in three years.

Organizations matter. Ensure buy-in and openness

Participants and authors alike describe from how important it was, throughout their deployment processes, to secure deep and widespread commitment and organizational buy-in, not just from eventual users but the partner organizations. This buy-in may be a particularly important point in health initiatives – it is rare for a new initiative to emerge and tackle green-field terrain. Systems must work well within or alongside existing public health administrations and procedures. In Lange's case in Chile, this meant that her team at the university had to spread and share credit for the diabetes management system with the Ministry of Health. Meanwhile, for MOTECH in Ghana, Osborn explains how the cooperation of the Ghana Health Service helped signal to nurses that the requirements of the system were part of their core jobs, not simply as 'something extra brought to them by an external organization that would one day go away'.

In the fishbowl session, these themes also surfaced, including linking with government ministries from the beginning to keep them involved throughout different phases of the project; aligning project data structures with those used by government; actively educating government ministries about the opportunities in mHealth, and working with local nongovernmental organizations to find out how best to align with government priorities and existing programs and systems.

Start with scale in mind. Decide if failure is an option

Peter Benjamin, a leader in mHealth for over ten years, expressed strong opinions about the push for scale in the mHealth field. 'Going from pilots to scale is really hard. Pilots are easier; there's a lot of attention, excitement, focus, more support.

To go to scale is really hard because almost the only way to plan is top down. It's much harder to get enthusiasm, energy in doing that.' Scale can be easier when working with telecommunications companies (Donner, Verclas and Toyama, 2008). In the fishbowl, one participant described how working with telecommunications companies can be arduous, with long approval processes and layers of meetings, but the scale (as Quraishi and Quraishi describe working with Reliance) is enormous. Partnerships can be achieved via corporate social responsibility (CSR) goals (as was the case with Text to Change in Uganda) or with the business development group, if the business case can be made. Osborn explained Grameen pursued this latter strategy with MTN in Ghana: 'Compared with working with the public sector, it's easier because you have similar goals, but financial sustainability is an issue.'

Regardless of telecommunications companies' involvement, an initiative's path to widespread adoption and use is likely to be a mix of serendipity, organic growth, and careful choices. As Gomez-Marquez explained in the fishbowl, starting with scale in mind is essential. Audience members echoed this point, drawing examples of both technical robustness and business models.

But there is some merit in pilots, and in caution. One related conversation brought some productive tension to the fishbowl. Some suggested that scale is not likely to be achieved through incremental tweaks to other pilots. Gomez-Marquez's comments and chapter reflect this perspective, suggesting that mHealth interventions may still be a place for thinking big, about 'high-risk, high reward' projects. 'Some will surely flop, but the winners might shine through' (or you might learn from failure itself – see http://failfaire.org). Another audience member, on the other hand, suggested that pursuing projects that might fail was irresponsible, since lives were at stake in health. A third attendee suggested rapid prototyping and solid testing, as a way to marry innovation with caution. Thus the facilitated dialogue brought participants toward a discussion of deeper assumptions and of change models, and made salient some difficulties in moving from pilot to scale. (If it were easy to move from pilot to scale, we would not see so many pilots that stay pilots.)

Local context matters

Similarly there was a tension between localism and scalability among the various projects and authors and finding the balance between localization and universality. This led to a range of decisions and trade-offs among the various approaches. For Divya Ramachandran this meant opting for a higher level of technology, namely videos featuring local women and health workers to strengthen the ability of the health worker to more effectively engage women in improved behaviors during pregnancy. 'When you think about content design – you need to be thinking behavior change, not about knowledge. We focused on two actions – saving money to prepare for an emergency during birth and ensuring women take iron.' It became increasingly necessary to identify what would motivate women to take up these two actions and to tailor the videos to such things, including dispelling myths about the effects of iron on babies.

In the case of Grameen, the findings of a formative ethnographic field study meant forgoing the original plan to use text messaging as part of their Mobile Midwife platform and direct to 'pregnant women' messaging to using voice recordings in local language and expanding the target audience to 'pregnant families' due to preferences for voice communication and shared mobile phones at the household level. Through the process of testing out voices and messages with local stakeholders, they were also able to refine and tailor messaging to appeal to their target audience.

For Text to Change, they found that partnering with local content experts and linking their program to local institutions provided familiarity and a direct mechanism for measuring the impact of their SMS-based quiz programs. In the case of Text to Change, they were able to assess the knowledge levels through the responses to their questions and at one point discovered that the questions were too easy – that they had to make them more challenging. They were also able to assess the impact of their messaging program in the uptake of HIV and AIDS testing and counseling services through their partnership with local service providers. According to Hajo van Beijma, 'as mHealth – we are trying to offer value to traditional health services.'

Link theory to practice via behavior change models

Linking theory to practice is common in academic settings. However, the notion of applying a change model to one's work was less familiar to some of the practitioners in the group. This was particularly felt throughout the iterative writing process, where many of the practitioners expressed some difficulties in articulating and aligning their assumptions with existing behavior change models – even though many of them subconsciously applied such models to the design of their platforms and programs. Many of the initiatives described in the book aim to increase awareness, knowledge, and self-efficacy; address beliefs, misconceptions, myths, and barriers; and introduce new behaviors, such as self-monitoring skills and adherence to medication in an effort to improve health outcomes and contribute to reduced costs, achieving Millennium Development Goals, and connecting the previously unreached. To generate change such programs aim to leverage social and peer pressure, beliefs, incentives, and competition. Persuasion was highlighted by Divya Ramachandran as a key driver of her work to target the beliefs that people have and build on them to catalyze change.

Very few of the participants in this process began with an explicit, articulated change theory – but rather focused on techniques that cut across multiple models or reflected post-haste on models that might apply to the choices they made in designing and implementing their programs. Games as a medium as in the case of ZMQ allow users the choice to create a virtual real-time scenario, quick learning, and behavior change through a hybrid approach that engages people in the use of social platforms into which people opt. Caroline Free's work on Text2Stop provides a recounting of the theoretical underpinnings of message creation and the mechanisms through which they ought to be delivered. In the private author discussions, many found kindred spirits in the challenges of formulating messages in a positive way with the appropriate tone, type, and amount of information.

The elusive art of measuring change

Given the desire to explore the range of approaches to evaluating the impact of mHealth on behavior change, we explicitly asked participants in both the external and internal dialogues to share their experiences in research and monitoring and evaluation. Heather Cole-Lewis's systematic review of SMS in disease prevention and disease management identified twelve studies for inclusion. Seven focused on disease management of which six were diabetes and one was asthma. Five studies focused on prevention, including one on smoking cessation and one on weight loss. All study designs included a measurable health outcome, but only nine had sufficient power to identify change (Cole-Lewis and Kershaw, 2010). For the others, there was consensus that it was very difficult to start with a research-driven approach as program design and the capabilities of what technology can do are changing rapidly. In addition, it was felt that within a few years of operation on the ground, the research questions change – making it a challenge to measure behavior change in a coherent manner.

For Divya Ramachandran it was felt that the 'evaluation process and design process need to be very linked – but it was hard to disaggregate how mHealth versus other interventions were affecting these expectant mothers.' According to Hajo van Beijma, it was difficult to start with a research-driven approach. Text2Change was engaged in three studies at the time of publication to help answer the question – *can we use social incentives to engage people in health programs?* Just a few years ago, people thought that technology could not change people's behaviors. A word of caution repeated frequently by Peter Benjamin is that 'counting SMSes is not evaluation. Things are starting to change and mHealth is becoming more legit.' Cell-Life will soon have data from two formal randomized control trials to answer the questions – *can cellphones support HIV+ mothers in Prevention of Mother to Child Transmission of HIV?* and *does sending SMSes to people change their behavior?*

Many people say that there is a psychological value in receiving SMSes. It makes them feel that the health system cares for them. We will know more when the study results come out.

Conclusion

This edited volume provides a platform for reflection and dialogue on an aspect of public health that has challenged practitioners for decades, namely behavior change. What happens then when from technology is introduced into the mix? There is a significant amount of hype and optimism surrounding mobile-mediated behavior change. This book aims to bring us down to earth to consider the collective experience of the pioneers who have learned by doing, some for over ten years. mHealth as a field is continuously evolving and platforms increasingly being mainstreamed and deployed at scale. Short of reinventing the wheel, the authors in this book provide insights that rarely see the light of day and couple them with the more academic and structured application of change models to better understand the pathways through which behavior change is possible.

Notes

1 General conference website: http://www.ictd2010.org.
Workshop website: http://www.mhealthybehaviors.org

2 http://failfaire.org

3 http://www.mhealthybehaviors.org

References

Amabile, T., Patterson, C., Mueller, J., Wojcik, T., Odomirok, P., Marsh, M. and Kramer, S. (2001), 'Academic-Practitioner Collaboration in Management Research: A Case of Cross-Profession Collaboration', *The Academy of Management Journal* 44(2): 418–31.

Argyris, C., Putnam, R. and Smith, D. (1985), *Action Science: Concepts, Methods and Skills for Research and Intervention*, San Francisco: Jossey-Bass.

Bakker, A. (2002), 'Health Care and ICT, Partnership Is a Must', *International Journal of Medical Informatics* 66(1-3): 51–7.

Cole-Lewis, H. and Kershaw, T. (2010), 'Text Messaging as a Tool for Behavior Change in Disease Prevention and Management', *Epidemiologic Reviews* 32(1): 56–69.

Donner, J. (2009), 'Mobile-Based Livelihood Services in Africa: Pilots and Early Deployments', in M. Fernandez-Ardevol and A. Ros (eds), *Communication Technologies in Latin America and Africa: A Multidisciplinary Perspective*, Barcelona: IN3: 37–58.

Fogg, B. and Adler, R. (2009), *Texting 4 Health: A Simple, Powerful Way to Change Lives*, Stanford: Captology Media.

Fogg, B. and Eckles, D. (2007), *Mobile Persuasion: 20 Perspectives of the Future of Behavior Change*, Stanford: Captology Media.

Frumkin, P. (2006), *Strategic Giving: The Art and Science of Philanthropy*, Chicago: University of Chicago Press.

Ginsburg, M. and Gorostiaga, J. (2001), 'Relationships between Theorists/Researchers and Policy Makers/Practitioners: Rethinking the Two-Cultures Thesis and the Possibility of Dialogue', *Comparative Education Review* 45(2): 173–96.

Heeks, R. (2002), 'Information Systems and Developing Countries: Failure, Success, and Local Improvisations', *The Information Society* 18(2): 101–12.

Hornick, R. ed. (2002), *Public Health Communication: Evidence for Behavior Change*. Mahwah, NJ, Lawrence Erlbaum.

Kantor, R. and Hoffman, L. (1966), 'Brechtian Theater as a Model for Conjoint Family Therapy', *Family Process* 5(2): 218–29.

Lefebvre, R. and Flora, J. (1988), 'Social Marketing and Public Health Intervention', *Health Education Behavior* 15(3): 299–315.

Lomas, J. (2007), 'The in-between World of Knowledge Brokering', *BMJ (Clinical research ed.)* 334(7585): 129–32.

Mechael, P., Batavia, H., Kaonga, N., Searle, S., Kwan, A., Fu, L. and Ossman, J. (2010), Barriers and Gaps Affecting mHealth in Low and Middle Income Countries: Policy White Paper. New York, Center for Global Health and Economic Development, Earth Institute, Columbia University.

Rice, R. and Atkin, C. eds., (2001), *Public Communication Campaigns*. Thousand Oaks, CA, Sage Publications, Inc.

Rice, R. and Katz, J. eds., (2001), *The Internet and Health Communication: Experiences and Expectations*. Thousand Oaks, CA, Sage Publications, Inc.

Schön, D. (1983), *The Reflective Practitioner: How Professionals Think in Action*, New York: Basic Books.

Siegel, M. and Lotenberg, L. (2004), *Marketing Public Health: Strategies to Promote Social Change*, Sudbury, MA: Jones and Bartlett.

Sjöberg, C. and Timpka, T. (1998), 'Participatory Design of Information Systems in Health Care', *JAMIA* 5: 177-83.

2 State of Behavior Change Initiatives and How Mobile Phones Are Transforming It

Ada Kwan, Mexican National Institute of Public Health, Patricia Mechael, mHealth Alliance at the UN Foundation and Earth Institute at Columbia University and Nadi Nina Kaonga, Earth Institute at Columbia University

Introduction

For many decades, public health interventions worldwide have utilized various strategies that can predict and modify the adoption and maintenance of healthier behaviors. At a time when the world's deadliest diseases are largely preventable and treatable, disease prevention is becoming increasingly emphasized, and behavior change has naturally become a central focus in public health. However, changing human behaviors and attitudes requires time, considerable effort, and motivation, and for those implementing programs, understanding the determinants of behavior can become ever more challenging.

In the past and present, different strategies have been employed to change behaviors or for persuasion. Successful interventions have used the following as vehicles to encourage people to be healthier: role models as examples of how to change, narratives with specific cultural and social links, personalized messages, and testimonials (Galavotti, Pappas-DeLuca and Lansky, 2001; Macintyre, Brown and Sosler, 2001). Knowing someone who is affected or has died of a related disease has also been a factor in changing behaviors. Reminders, cues, prompts, and incentives are additional ways to modify behavior, and they have been spread through mediums such as radio, television, and other forms of mass media (Elder, 2001).

More recently, mobile technologies have exploded in popularity, unlocking a unique vehicle for eliciting behavior change. With nearly 5.3 billion mobile phone subscriptions worldwide at the end of 2010, the ubiquity of mobile phones and networks is providing countless opportunities for health behavior change initiatives in high-, middle-, and low-income countries (ITU, 2010). Within these initiatives, mobile phones are being used for every stage of disease – from health knowledge and promotion to disease prevention, diagnosis, and treatment, including appointment reminders and medication compliance. However, the application of mobile phones in health behavior change interventions does not stop there, as their abilities to link to software applications and back-end systems can make data collection possible, medical records more electronic and up to date, and patient–provider relationships stronger (Mechael *et al.* 2010). On an organizational level, mobile technologies are offering an opportunity for individuals to communicate comfortably without being in the same physical space (Kegler and Glanz, 2008).

Although mobile phones have been the focus of thorough and advanced research in developed countries (Fogg and Eckles, 2007; Fogg and Adler, 2009), what we know about mobile phones and behavior change mechanisms is less known among less-developed countries. Additionally, not only do we need to further understand existing factors and processes that can elicit behavior change, we need to more importantly and pragmatically understand strategies that should exist. In five parts, this introduction will describe the state of mHealth, or the use of mobile phones for health, in behavior change initiatives and research in low- and middle-income countries: (1) a snapshot of mobile-mediated behavior change projects; (2) health promotion and disease prevention; (3) disease management, treatment compliance, and appointment reminders; (4) theory in mHealth behavior change initiatives; and (5) a reflection on what 'mobile' brings to the behavior change world and what more there is to understand.

Snapshot of mHealth behavior change interventions

In general, mHealth behavior change initiatives focus on the spectrum of disease and illness with different target populations. In this section, we paint the landscape of mHealth behavior change through brief responses to the following questions:

- What kinds of mHealth behavior change projects exist in LMICs?
- How do social, cultural, and political contexts play a role?
- What can mobile phones provide?
- How are mobile phones utilized to change behavior?
- How do these projects begin and to whom do they target?

Figure 2.1 displays a variety of mobile-mediated behavior change projects in LMICs. The figure and the descriptions that follow (and more examples will be introduced throughout this book) are by no means intended to be representative

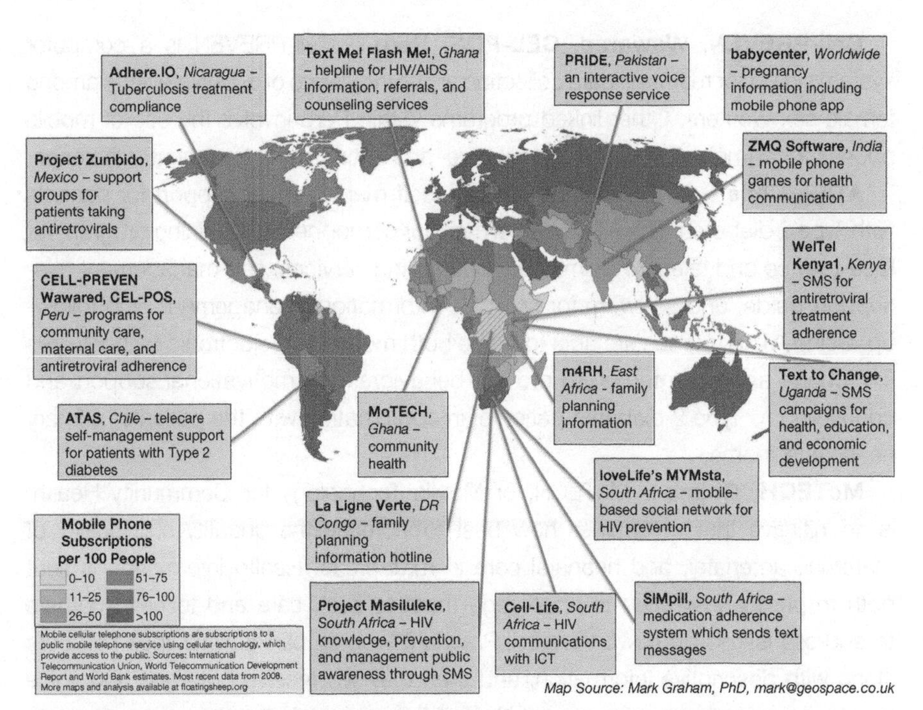

Figure 2.1 mHealth behavior change projects

Source: Highlights of mHealth behavior change interventions on a world map displaying 2008 mobile phone subscriptions per 100 people by country (permission granted to use and alter map entitled 'Map of per-capita mobile phone subscriptions' by Mark Graham, PhD. (Graham, 2011)).

but should instead reflect projects that collectively demonstrate several approaches for mobile-led behavior change.

What kinds of mHealth behavior change projects exist in LMICs?

Below is a brief description for each of the projects included in Figure 2.1.

Adhere.IO Nicaragua – Individuals in a tuberculosis program are incentivized to achieve high treatment compliance rates with mobile minutes or credit. Program participants are given urinalysis test strips dispensed every twenty-four hours. These strips contain four numbers and embedded chemicals, which react with urine from patients who have properly taken their TB medication. Patients then send a text message reporting the numbers on the strip, and those with high compliance rates are rewarded.

Project Zumbido, Mexico – Project Zumbido created a mobile phone support group for patients taking antiretroviral medications. Within three months of the pilot, 25,000 text messages were sent among the forty participants, who also sent voice messages and participated in conference calls. Support and information were exchanged, which encouraged the patients to better monitor their disease.

Cell-PREVEN, Wawared, CEL-POS, Peru – Cell-PREVEN is a computer system set up for real-time data collection and surveillance of adverse events among female sex workers. Other linked programs within Peru involve the use of mobile phones for community care, maternal care, and antiretroviral treatment adherence.

ATAS, Chile – ATAS provides telecare, self-management support for patients with Type 2 diabetes. The ATAS model has four components: a training program for face-to-face and telecare teams; tele-counseling services; self-management tele-support guide; and software for self-care information, management, and follow-up. Using ATAS, nurses are able to utilize both mobile and electronic technologies (i.e. phone and the internet) to provide behavioral and motivational support and counseling to Type 2 diabetes patients, in coordination with the patients' primary healthcare teams.

MoTECH, Ghana – MoTECH, or Mobile Technology for Community Health, is an initiative that determines how best to increase the quantity and quality of maternal, antenatal, and neonatal care in rural areas. Health information is sent both to pregnant women to encourage them to seek care and to new mothers to address issues on newborn care. Pregnant women can register their numbers along with descriptive information, and then they will receive both text and voice messages regarding pregnancy, health facilities, and treatments.

Text Me! Flash Me!, Ghana – Connecting individuals to a helpline for HIV/AIDS information, referrals, and counseling services, Text Me! Flash Me! also sends text messages containing information collected from ongoing quality assurance and monitoring and evaluation information. Text Me! posters are created to inform the public of the service and that texting specific HIV-related words to a number allows users to receive more information about the texted topic. The Flash Me! component offers a strategy for individuals to flash a helpline counselor, who can then return the call within twenty-four hours, making the call free for the inquirer.

La Ligne Verte, DR Congo – To respond to a lack of knowledge in family planning products and services, the toll-free family planning hotline La Ligne Verte was created in 2005. Mobile phone operators Vodacom and Zain set up the hotline, which was paid by Population Services International and its local affiliate Association de Santé Familiale. The hotline operated between the hours of 8:00 a.m. to 4:30 p.m., and in its first four years, the hotline received 80,000 calls from across the country. Interestingly, the hotline was originally targeted to women of reproductive age; however, approximately 80 percent of the callers were male. This may suggest a strong unmet demand for family-planning-related knowledge for men.

Project Masiluleke, South Africa – 'Project M' is encouraging the general public to get tested for HIV, alerting patients to take their antiretroviral medications, and providing support for self-testing all by leveraging the features of mobile phones. The launch of the project included the daily delivery of approximately one million 'Please Call Me' text messages for one year. A free form of text messaging, these messages linked users to HIV call centers, and the campaign tripled average call volumes to the National AIDS Helpline in Johannesburg.

Cell-Life, South Africa – Cell-Life is using text message reminders for improving treatment adherence and providing information to empower individuals to choose risk-reducing behavior among its long list of activities that involve communicating many HIV topics with mobile phones. Topics include mass messaging for prevention, mass information for positive living, linking patients and clinics, peer-to-peer support and counseling, building organizational capacity of HIV-related organizations, and monitoring and evaluation.

SIMpill, South Africa – SIMpill is a medication adherence system that alerts patients and caregivers through text messages when medication has not been taken. The technology has been used to remind TB patients to take their medication. The bottle is outfitted with a SIM card and transmitter. Each time the bottle is opened, an SMS is sent to a server. If the bottle is not opened when it should be, a notification is sent to the patient and/or their caregiver.

loveLife's MYMsta, South Africa – loveLife's MYMsta is a social network that harnesses the features of mobile phones to spread HIV prevention information, in addition to bursary information and employment opportunities to South African youths.

m4RH, East Africa – A service that sends family planning information via text messages, m4RH can be accessed after individuals send a text message containing 'm4RH' to a specific number. The individuals then receive a list of topics, such as contraceptive information or family planning clinic locations. The different options can be entered as a reply, and the individual is then able to access these different options.

Text to Change, Uganda – Although initiated in Uganda, Text to Change's SMS campaigns for health, education, and economic development can now be found across Africa, as well as other countries in the world. The organization's health education programs, aimed to be interactive and incentive-based, encourage testing and drug compliance and inform people of options of which they may or may not be aware regarding health services.

WelTel Kenya1, Kenya – Implemented by an organization that uses evidence to improve strategic planning of health interventions, WelTel Kenya1 was a randomized controlled trial (RCT) evaluating the use of SMS for antiretroviral treatment adherence.

ZMQ Software, India – ZMQ Software considers mobile phone games as a method to learn about health topics. In India, one of the projects provides information through SMS to women about prenatal care. As of 2009, nearly 18,000 women had participated in this program by enrolling their numbers at hospitals; however, ZMQ is trying to offer women the opportunity to enroll directly by sending an SMS.

PRIDE, Pakistan – The PRIDE project has been using mobile technologies to increase access to maternal and child health information and services. Initiatives include interactive voice response (IVR) services and text message reminders for antenatal care, immunizations, and post-natal care.

BabyCenter, Worldwide – In addition to being a source of information for expecting mothers, BabyCenter offers two services on mobile phones. BabyCenter's Booty Caller offers a series of eighteen text message ovulation alerts, and BabyCenter Mobile provides expecting mothers advice on pregnancies. Recently, in collaboration with the Grameen Foundation, BabyCenter has been working on a mobile-phone-based fundraising and education campaign for pregnant women to learn more about their pregnancies, in addition to advice on avoiding malaria and managing pregnancy-related costs.

How do social, cultural, and political contexts play a role?

In these projects, social, cultural, and political contexts play a large role not only in the feasibility and perceptions of using mobile phones or other information and communication technologies, but also in each stage of the project. Thus, getting to know the target audience is of great importance. Considerations must also be made for resource-limited contexts. For example, populations in which illiteracy rates are high are likely to not benefit from a text messaging program. For the populations where a text messaging program is feasible, specific words and phrases may be of much more influence than others, and it is up to program implementers and all stakeholders to determine what combination of words will be the most successful in inducing healthier behaviors.

Exploring the acceptability and perceptions among individuals to use mobile phones and their features as a medium to deliver health promotion or treatment reminders in a useful and culturally specific way has seen increasing efforts in recent years, resulting in growing evidence. It was found that among HIV-positive individuals in Peru, just under one quarter were already informally using alarms on their mobile phones as reminders to take their medications, and others found alarm reminders to be necessary (Curioso and Kurth, 2007). Individuals also expressed a desire to receive information via their mobile phones on their personal sexual health, general information on sexually transmitted infections (STIs), general HIV information, recent advances in HIV treatment, and up-to-date research. Compared with in-person interactions, individuals also found mobile phones to offer greater confidentiality. At a community-based clinic in Lima, Peru, patients expressed the importance of messages to be confidential and private (e.g. by using 'coded' words, such as '*Remember, it is the time of your life*'), as well as be written in simple and concise words (Curioso, Quistberg, Cabello, Gozzer, Garcia, Holmes, and Kurth, 2009).

What can mobile phones provide?

In addition to differing in social, cultural, and political contexts, projects differ by the particular mobile phone features utilized to elicit behavior change. Varying across mobile phone models, features include voice, text, multimedia messaging service (for example picture and video messaging), and applications, such as camera, calendar, and the internet. One of the most used features across phones, as well as for behavior change, is text messaging, also known as short message service (SMS). In a review of twenty-five studies selected solely to demonstrate the use of voice and text features on mobile phones conducted in 2009, eight projects used voice and SMS; another eight projects combined the internet with SMS; and the remaining nine utilized SMS only (Krishna, Boren and Balas, 2009).

How are mobile phones utilized to change behavior?

In mobile-mediated behavior change projects, attempts to elicit desired behavior changes can be simply from created to either directly or indirectly target a desired change, which can be a reduction of a behavior related to poor health or an increase of a behavior related to better health. Examples of these forms of behavior change include:

- Direct way to reduce behavior related to poor health:
    - Text messages to encourage an individual to stop smoking
- Indirect way to reduce behavior related to poor health:
    - Information about how to effectively stop smoking
    - Information about lung cancer statistics to encourage smoking cessation
- Direct way to increase behavior related to better health:
    - Text messages to remind HIV/AIDS patients to take antiretroviral medication
    - Text messages to encourage exercise
- Indirect way to increase behavior related to better health:
    - Information about available HIV and STI hotlines
    - Information for pregnant women regarding mother and newborn care from pregnancy to after birth

When categorizing the mHealth projects in Figure 2.1 in this fashion, the majority of the projects focus on increasing behavior related to better health in both direct and indirect ways. Additionally, we see that mHealth efforts distinctly increase behaviors that prevent or mitigate infectious diseases, primarily HIV/AIDS and other STIs, or promote behaviors to improve maternal and child health. In higher income countries HICs, where chronic diseases are the main killers, mHealth efforts focus more often than not on increasing or reducing behaviors linked to the development of chronic diseases, such as exercise to prevent or mitigate heart disease, and smoking cessation to prevent or mitigate lung disease, respectively. Although the primary purpose of this book is to introduce behavior change efforts in the mobile phone era of LMICs, it is important to draw some lessons learned from HICs as the epidemiological profiles of LMICs reflect shifting disease burdens from infectious diseases to chronic diseases. From the review of the twenty-five studies, which happened to draw from studies in high and upper-middle income countries, described above, ten were related to evaluating behavior change outcomes, such as smoking cessation (reducing smoking behaviors) and antiretroviral (ARV) treatment adherence (increasing proper medication intake behaviors), and the majority of studies concluded that information and knowledge delivered through mobile phones could result in clinical health and health process improvements.

How do these projects begin and to whom do they target?

mHealth behavior change projects generally spawn from supply or demand. In 2009, Fjeldsoe, Marshall and Miller *et al.* performed a review of fourteen studies on health behavior change interventions delivered by text messaging. Out of these fourteen studies, 29 percent (n = 4) targeted health behavior change in prevention, and the remaining 71 percent (n = 10) targeted health behavior change in clinical care. Text messages in each of the prevention interventions were 'research-initiated'; those in most of the clinical care interventions were 'participant-initiated', where initiation refers to the body that initiated the dialogue via text messages. Very few of the interventions were theory-based, and the authors suggest that behavior change theory should be described more explicitly in future studies (more detail on theory later on). Twelve of the studies sent patients tailored messages, which incorporated the participant's name or nickname, nominated support person's name, age, gender, behavioral history, behavioral preferences, behavioral goals, behavioral barriers, previous text message responses, and medical status (Fjeldsoe *et al.*, 2009). Interestingly, the two studies using untailored messages were in the top three for highest participant attrition. Eight of the studies the authors reviewed reported significant and positive behavioral change, and an additional five had positive behavior trends that were not significantly significant. The authors mention that there is a strong attempt in research to measure outcomes objectively; however, the effects of targeted behavior are lacking in the literature. Additionally, because most studies reflected pilots or feasibility tests, sample sizes were relatively small to provide sufficient statistical power. The authors suggest future studies should use larger sample sizes.

Health promotion and disease prevention

Regarding health promotion and disease prevention, mobile phones are delivering interventions to promote and disseminate information for sex, family planning, and STIs, particularly HIV, and to encourage individuals to stop smoking and lose weight, respectively. Aimed at improving health behaviors and psychological and physical symptoms, interventions using palm computers or mobile phones can be successfully delivered, are accepted by patients, and are efficacious for treating a wide variety of health behaviors and physical and psychological symptoms (Heron and Smyth, 2010).

For encouraging and reinforcing health behaviors, text messages are frequently employed as an effective strategy; however, they should not be considered stand-alone for behavior change, but as a tool by which behavior change methods can be administered (Cole-Lewis and Kershaw, 2010). Whether or not these projects are effective can only be deduced from robust evaluations, which require sufficient time and support for implementation and monitoring and evaluation. In their review of literature for text messaging in disease prevention and management, Cole-Lewis and Kershaw assessed seventeen articles that reported on twelve studies (one conducted in a developing country) where interventions ranged from three to twelve months (Cole-Lewis and Kershaw, 2010). Three of the twelve studies were inconclusive, and eight of nine powered studies found evidence that text messaging for disease prevention and management was effective. A review was also conducted for mHealth text messaging interventions for sexual health education and management (Lim, Hocking, Hellard, and Aitken, 2008). Evidence appeared to be lacking on the effectiveness of these programs (the authors provided the goals, context, and potential of these programs); however, only one RCT was known among these programs.

Demonstrating how physical activity can be increased through text messaging, an RCT was conducted on the physical activity intervention called MobileMums. Eighty-eight postnatal women were randomized into a control or intervention group (Fjeldsoe, Miller and Marshall, 2010). The control group did not receive any contact or resources aside from a telephone reminder to confirm their week six and week thirteen assessments, whereas the intervention group received two physical activity goal setting consultations with a behavioral counselor (one in-person and one over the telephone), a refrigerator magnet for planning weekly activities and monitoring physical activity goals and rewards, forty-two (three to five SMSes a week) text messages with personally tailored messages with behavioral and cognitive approaches, eleven weekly text messages sufficing as 'goal checks', and instructions for selecting someone to assist the participant in reaching activity goals. On average, the intervention group increased physical activity by 1.82 days/week and walking for exercise by 1.08 days/week. The participants described the magnet to be the 'most helpful component' for changing their behavior.

The growth of health hotlines has also been observed with the potential of mobile phones to spread information on conditions of interest for individuals. In the Democratic Republic of Congo, the program La Ligne Verte ('hotline' in French) offers individuals an opportunity to speak with those trained in high-quality family planning and contraceptive information and in making referrals to clinics if needed (PSI DR Congo and Toth, 2008). Most interestingly, although women were the target population for the family planning information, 80 per cent of callers have been men of reproductive age, perhaps reflecting an unmet demand for such information (PSI DR Congo and Toth, 2008). Additionally, Ivatury and colleagues looked at different health hotlines in Bangladesh, Pakistan, India, and Mexico that together provided information to over ten million individuals, mostly women in rural areas (Mechael, Batavia, Kaonga, Searle, Kwan, Fu, and Ossman, 2010). Not only are hotlines a 'reliable and supportive source of help', but they offer an opportunity to overcome barriers such as limited numbers of healthcare workers to meet with patients and costs in time and money for unnecessary transportation to clinics (Mechael *et al.*, 2010).

Disease management, treatment compliance, and appointment reminders

For individuals who are living with diseases, mobile phones are being utilized in behavior change interventions for disease management, drug adherence, and appointment reminders. As mentioned earlier, projects in HICs heavily focus on the management of chronic diseases, and projects in LMICs heavily focus on the management of infectious diseases, particularly HIV/AIDS. Interventions are primarily delivered through text messages, followed by voice, web browsers, and health hotlines (Mechael *et al.*, 2010).

Users of a clinic in both urban and rural south India were asked about their mobile phone usage behaviors and other topics considered to be important for designing a mobile phone based intervention for ARV treatment adherence (Shet, Arumugam, Rodrigues, Rajagopalan, Shubha, Raj, D'souza, and De Costa, 2010). Ownership was lower in rural settings, but still a majority of users (60 percent) mentioned that the 'most acceptable intervention' would be automated voice calls, opposed to text messages, at a weekly frequency, opposed to a daily frequency. One caveat to this is that the users of the clinic may actually respond much differently to the way they mentioned when asked. In other words, 'perceived responses do not automatically translate to actual behaviors' (Shet *et al.*, 2010).

For improving appointment attendance, SMS reminders have been shown to be successful; however, a handful of other studies found mixed results, and others with small samples were inconclusive (Mechael *et al.*, 2010). One RCT in Cote d'Ivoire evaluated text messages for improving malaria chemoprophylaxis adherence among French soldiers (n = 424) (Ollivier, Romand, Marimoutou, Michel, Pognant, Todesco, Migliani, Baudon, and Boutin, 2009). Although cited as being useful by the treatment group, the text messages did not significantly improve adherence, but overall treatment adherence was higher than expected. One possible explanation and limitation of the study was that soldiers in treatment and control groups were in close enough contact to remind each other when to take the medications, which could have caused a weakened measured effect between the two groups.

Within the literature, many RCTs on the use of mobile phones for ARV treatment are emerging from LMICs – providing more clues to what may be effective in certain contexts. In an RCT with 538 participants randomized into a treatment group receiving text messages and a control group receiving standard care in Kenya, HIV patients who received text messages had ARV treatment adherence rates that were significantly higher than those in the control group (Lester, Rivto, Mills, Kariri, Karanja, Chung, Jack, Habyarimana, Sadatsafavi, Najafzadeh, Marra, Estambale, Ngugi, Ball, Thabane, Gelmon, Kimani, Ackers, and Plummer 2010). These increases in adherence rates among patients in the treatment group were confirmed by significant increases in rates of viral suppression. Also in Kenya, 431 adult patients who had recently begun ARV treatment for HIV were randomized into a control group or one of four intervention groups, which received either short or long text messages sent at a daily or weekly frequency. Short messages were designed to determine whether a simple reminder was sufficient to change behavior; long messages, whether additional support was more effective. Daily messages were sent at a frequency close to proper treatment usage, and weekly messages sent to avoid the possibility of too frequent messages becoming habituating. Weekly reminders improved the amount of patients having achieved 90 percent ARV treatment adherence.

Theory in mHealth behavior change initiatives

As the uptake of mobile phones strongly offers a new strategy for the field of behavior change, it will be important to attentively assess the integration of this new strategy within existing and/or new theories. This is extremely important because behavior change is hard to do for different reasons, such as varying levels of motivation in individuals who are targeted for behavior change interventions, in combination with the difficulty in reducing an unhealthy behavior that makes an individual feel good, such as smoking, or increasing a behavior that an individual already has begun to an extent versus an individual who has not begun that behavior. Messaging interventions that are designed and evaluated based on theory have been found to be more successful, and theory is being applied more frequently in some disease interventions than in others (Cole-Lewis and Kershaw, 2010; Riley, Rivera, Atienza, Nilsen, Allison, and Mermelstein, 2011). When reviewing fourteen studies on text messaging health behavior change interventions, Fjeldsoe et al. found four studies that were implemented through a theoretical basis (Fjeldsoe and Kershaw 2009). Theories applied included social cognitive theory, behavioral self-regulation theory, relapse prevention, and a combination of social psychological theories. The authors suggest that the stronger focus on behavior change in clinical care compared with preventive care may be a reason for fewer studies providing a theoretical basis. In another systematic review of literature on mobile health interventions, Riley *et al.* found that most smoking and weight loss studies reported a theoretical basis and that most of the adherence and chronic disease (for example, diabetes, asthma, and hypertension) management studies did not (Riley *et al.*, 2011). Among the seven smoking prevention, twelve weight-loss, ten treatment adherence, and twenty chronic disease management mHealth interventions, the authors found that those interventions based on theory drew most frequently from, in decreasing order, health belief model, theory of planned behavior, social cognitive theory, transtheoretical theory, self-determination theory, self-efficacy theory, and contingent theory. It appears as though deeper applications of theory across mobile health behavior interventions will have strong benefits, but existing theories lack the qualities or constructs that can fully inform development. In this regard, it is likely that mobile phone integration into health behavior interventions will push theory development, particularly as these systems become more dynamic, adaptive, and interactive (Riley *et al.*, 2011).

Reflection on what 'Mobile' brings to the behavior change world – reach, access, and mobility

Mobile phones have become attractive vehicles for delivering behavior change interventions (Mechael *et al.*, 2010). We are currently seeing mobile phones relay information, send encouragement, and provide reminders, as well as make available contact information for hotlines, counseling, and educators along the cascade of health services provided in LMICs. In this section, we reflect on what mobile phones have brought to the behavior change world.

Mobile phones have become so ubiquitous in recent years, particularly because of flexible payment plans, that they provide an unmet opportunity for reaching and accessing neglected populations (Mechael *et al.*, 2010). From a public health perspective, behavior change interventions ought to be delivered with equitable access, and mobile phones, having reached all corners of the world and all socioeconomic and education levels, offer a huge advantage over traditional health behavior change techniques (for example radio, landline telephones, and the internet) to reach more disadvantaged groups of the population who are less likely to have access to health interventions while being the ones who may need it the most (Fjeldsoe *et al.*, 2010).

The fact that mobile phones are cheap, small, and can be personal offers individuals communication flexibility with features, namely voice calls and text messaging, through which health professionals can create a more interactive way to promote health, prevent disease or illness, and manage disease and treatments (Cole-Lewis and Kershaw, 2010). For promoting health, text messages are quick and immediate vehicles for tasks such as carrying information about family planning (PSI DR Congo and Toth, 2008) and quizzes about HIV/AIDS knowledge and beliefs (Henriquez, 2009). For preventing disease, health professionals are primarily using voice call strategies and text messaging for encouraging individuals to exercise more and stop smoking (Krishna *et al.*, 2009). For disease management and treatment, simple text messages are being utilized as reminders for patients to take their medications (Lester *et al.*, 2010; Pop-Eleches, Thirumurthy, Habyarimana, Zivin, Goldstein, de Walque, MacKeen, Haberer, Kimaiyo, Sidle, Ngare, and Bangsberg, 2011). Low start-up costs of these interventions, the ability to use existing infrastructure (mobile networks), and, as previously mentioned, the potential of mobile phones to run software applications and link to back-end systems offer additional advantages (Lester *et al.*, 2010; Mechael *et al.*, 2010). To summarize, many of these strategies exhibit opportunities for individuals to self-manage their health and to take ownership of their health while receiving real-time or close-to-real-time responses or feedback (Suter, Suter and Johnston, 2011). In many ways, interaction through mobile phones is affording new possibilities in behavior change: for some interventions, existing communication channels are being strengthened, and for others, new communication channels are being created to induce healthier behavior.

More specifically, as a promising vehicle for health behavior change intervention delivery, the ability of text messaging to offer reminders or bits of encouragement may tap important constructs central to many behavioral theories, such as cues to action, reinforcement, and social support (Cole-Lewis and Kershaw, 2010). Other features of text messaging that allow it to be a strong tool for healthcare improvement include its availability on almost every model of mobile phones, relatively low cost, widespread use, no requirements for great technological expertise, asynchronous (for example, if the phone is turned off, messages can be delivered when the phone is turned back on, or if the battery dies or the power is lost, messages can be received when the battery is recharged or when the power returns), and access of messages at any time. These features allow mobile phones to be widely applicable to a variety of health behaviors and conditions, as well as in-the-moment, personally tailored health communication reinforcement (Cole-Lewis and Kershaw, 2010).

There is more to understand on what 'Mobile' can bring to behavior change

Among the aforementioned, there is more to understand on what mobile phones can bring to behavior change. First, rigorous evaluations of mHealth behavior change interventions are the exception and not the rule. Much of the existing research findings are from pilot or feasibility studies, which have small sample sizes or not enough power to identify significance across intervention and nonintervention groups. This makes it even more difficult to conclude what particular behavior mechanisms are in play when an individual finds, for example, encouragement from text messages to exercise more or to go get tested for STIs at the nearest clinic. To further understand the determinants of behavior change, scale up is necessary for some of these programs, which could benefit very much from strong private–public partnerships among donors, program managers, ministries of health, evaluation teams, mobile phone companies, healthcare professionals, and those targeted to receive the interventions (Lester *et al.*, 2010; Mechael *et al.*, 2010). Second, most of the health behavior change interventions are delivered via SMS, which presents the issue that illiterate members of a population cannot be included in a text messaging intervention, perhaps a reason why interventions that target populations with higher rates of illiteracy are known to use voice features, such as interactive voice response systems. This has previously been suggested as the 'rate-limiting step on use of text messaging' (Kaplan, 2006). Third, the mobile phone will be a channel for triggering many behaviors (Fogg and Adler, 2009), but it is important to consider the inability to send tailored messages to an individual in a context where mobile phones are often shared, usually among household members. In the case where someone is borrowing another person's phone, calls and texts can be sent but perhaps not received, whereas the person who owns the phone can both send and receive phone calls and text messages (James and Versteeg, 2007). Fourth, generalizability across different populations, across different times, or across different diseases or illnesses can be fallacious. Similarly, as exhibited by the evolution of behavior change models and their applications in different settings, a model created and meant for use in an HIC may not be suitable for use in a low-income country, or vice versa (Bertrand, 2004; Kaplan, 2006). Similarly, existing research conducted in HICs corresponds to chronic diseases, and research conducted in LMIC settings generally correspond to infectious diseases, mostly HIV/AIDS-related. This brings up two issues: (1) Findings from these studies may not be generalizable to other diseases or illnesses or from one setting to the next, so reapplying findings from one study to a new context is cautioned, and (2) As LMICs are currently facing epidemiologic transitions, the application of health behavior change interventions, especially those for prevention, targeting chronic diseases are just as important as those targeting infectious diseases. However, successful mHealth behavior interventions can provide invaluable knowledge, as well as a skeleton and platform upon which additional behavioral interventions for other diseases or illnesses can be introduced. Although the list of what mobile phones can provide to the field of behavior change is extensive, it is matched with an even more extensive list of what there is to learn. In order to reach the full potential of mHealth behavior change, it will be crucial to understand these.

Closing

We hope that this introduction has provided sufficient background information on behavior change interventions in the context of nearly saturated global mobile phone uptake. Through a snapshot of mHealth behavior change projects, we briefly touched upon a handful of projects taking place in LMICs, which reflect mobile phone strategies in health promotion and disease prevention to disease management, treatment compliance, and appointment reminders. We have touched on theory in these initiatives, and how interventions designed and evaluated based on theory have been found to be more successful. All in all, mobile phones provide reach, access, and mobility to the field of behavior change, but there is a lot more to learn before full potential can be possible. In the next chapters, this book will provide a deeper look into several of these interventions across the world.

Bibliography

Bertrand, J. (2004), 'Diffusion of Innovations and HIV/AIDS', *Journal of Health Communication* 9: 113–21.

Cole-Lewis, H. and Kershaw, T. (2010), 'Text Messaging as a Tool for Behavior Change in Disease Prevention and Management', *Epidemiologic Reviews* 32(1): 56–69.

Curioso, W. and Kurth, A. (2007), 'Access, Use and Perceptions Regarding Internet, Cell Phones and PDAs as a Means for Health Promotion for People Living with HIV in Peru', *BMC Medical Informatics and Decision Making* 7(24).

Curioso, W., Quistberg, D., Cabello, R., Gozzer, E., Garcia, P., Holmes, K. and Kurth, A. (2009), '"It's Time for Your Life": How Should We Remind Patients to Take Medicine Using Short Text Messages?', *AMIA Annual Symposium Proceedings*: 129–33.

Elder, J. (2001), *Behavior Change and Public Health in the Developing World*, Thousand Oaks: Sage Publications.

Fjeldsoe, B., Marshall, A. and Miller, Y. (2009), 'Behavior Change Interventions Delivered by Mobile Telephone Short-Message Service', *American Journal of Preventive Medicine* 36(2): 165–73.

Fjeldsoe, B., Miller, Y. and Marshall, A. (2010), 'MobileMums: A Randomized Controlled Trial of an SMS-Based Physical Activity Intervention', *Annals of Behavioral Medicine* 39: 101–11.

Fogg, B. and Adler, R. (2009), *Texting 4 Health: A Simple, Powerful Way to Change Lives*, Stanford: Captology Media.

Fogg, B. and Eckles, D. (2007), *Mobile Persuasion: 20 Perspectives of the Future of Behavior Change*, Stanford: Captology Media.

Galavotti, C., Pappas-DeLuca, K. and Lansky, A. (2001), 'Modeling and Reinforcement to Combat HIV: The March Approach to Behavior Change', *American Journal of Public Health* 91(10): 1602–7.

Graham, M. (2011), 'Map of Per-Capita Mobile Phone Subscriptions', http://www.floatingsheep.org/2011/01/map-of-per-capita-mobile-phone.html [Accessed 15 February 2012].

Henriquez, K. (2009), 'Text to Change: Spreading the Message to Stop the Virus', http://ict4uganda.wordpress.com/2009/03/31/text-to-change-spreading-the-message-to-stop-the-virus/ [Accessed 15 February 2012].

Heron, K. and Smyth, J. (2010), 'Ecological Momentary Interventions: Incorporating Mobile Technology into Psychosocial and Health Behavior Treatments', *British Journal of Health Psychology* 15(Part 1): 1–39.

ITU. (2010), 'Measuring the Information Society', http://www.itu.int/pub/D-IND-ICTOI-2010/en [Accessed 15 February 2012].

Ivatury, G., Moore, J. and Bloch, A. (2009), 'A Doctor in Your Pocket: Health Hotlines in Developing Countries', *Innovations: Technology, Governance, Globalization* 4(1): 119–53.

James, J. and Versteeg, M. (2007), 'Mobile Phones in Africa: How Much Do We Really Know?', *Social Indicators Research* 84: 117–26.

Kaplan, W. (2006), 'Can the Ubiquitous Power of Mobile Phones Be Used to Improve Health Outcomes in Developing Countries?', *Globalization and Health* 2: 9.

Kegler, M. and Glanz, K. (2008), 'Perspectives on Group, Organization, and Community Interventions', in K. Glanz, B. Rimer and K. Viswanath (eds), *Health Behavior and Health Education: Theory, Research, and Practice*, San Francisco: Jossey-Bass: 389–404.

Krishna, S., Boren, S. and Balas, E. (2009), 'Healthcare Via Cell Phones: A Systematic Review', *Telemedicine and e-Health* 15(3): 231–41.

Lester, R., Rivto, P., Mills, E., Kariri, A., Karanja, S., Chung, M., Jack, W., Habyarimana, J., Sadatsafavi, M., Najafzadeh, M., Marra, C., Estambale, B., Ngugi, E., Ball, T., Thabane, L., Gelmon, L., Kimani, J., Ackers, M. and Plummer, F. (2010), 'Effects of a Mobile Phone Short Message Service on Antiretroviral Treatment Adherence in Kenya (Weltel Kenya1): A Randomised Trial', *Lancet* 376(9755): 1838–45.

Lim, M., Hocking, J., Hellard, M. and Aitken, C. (2008), 'SMS STI: A Review of the Uses of Mobile Phone Text Messaging in Sexual Health', *International Journal of STD & AIDS* 19: 287–90.

Macintyre, K., Brown, L. and Sosler, S. (2001), '"It's Not What You Know, but Who You Knew": Examining the Relationship between Behavior Change and AIDS Mortality in Africa', *AIDS Education and Prevention* 13(2): 160–74.

Mechael, P., Batavia, H., Kaonga, N., Searle, S., Kwan, A., Fu, L. and Ossman, J. (2010), Barriers and Gaps Affecting mHealth in Low and Middle Income Countries: Policy White Paper. New York, Center for Global Health and Economic Development, Earth Institute, Columbia University.

Ollivier, L., Romand, O., Marimoutou, C., Michel, R., Pognant, C., Todesco, A., Migliani, R., Baudon, D. and Boutin, J. (2009), 'Use of Short Message Service (SMS) to Improve Malaria Chemoprophylaxis Compliance after Returning from a Malaria Endemic Area', *Malaria Journal* 8(236).

Pop-Eleches, C., Thirumurthy, H., Habyarimana, J., Zivin, J., Goldstein, M., de Walque, D., MacKeen, L., Haberer, J., Kimaiyo, S., Sidle, J., Ngare, D. and Bangsberg, D. (2011), 'Mobile

Phone Technologies Improve Adherence to Antiretroviral Treatment in a Resource-Limited Setting: A Randomized Controlled Trial of Text Message Reminders', *AIDS* 25(6): 825–34.

PSI DR Congo and Toth, C. (2008), 'Cell Phone Hotline Spreads Family Planning Information in DR Congo', Washington, DC: USAID. www.flexfund.org/resources/technical_updates/psi_drc_case_study.pdf [Accessed 15 February 2012].

Riley, W., Rivera, D., Atienza, A., Nilsen, W., Allison, S. and Mermelstein, R. (2011), 'Health Behavior Models in the Age of Mobile Interventions: Are Our Theories up to the Task?', *Translational Behavioral Medicine* 1(1): 53–71.

Shet, A., Arumugam, K., Rodrigues, R., Rajagopalan, N., Shubha, K., Raj, T., D'souza, G. and De Costa, A. (2010), 'Designing a Mobile Phone-Based Intervention to Promote Adherence to Antiretroviral Therapy in South India', *AIDS and Behavior* 14(3): 716–20.

Suter, P., Suter, W. and Johnston, D. (2011), 'Theory-Based Telehealth and Patient Empowerment', *Population Health Management* 14(2): 1–8.

3 mHealthy Behavior Studies

Lessons from a systematic review

Heather Cole-Lewis, Yale School of Public Health

Background

In early 2010, my article entitled 'Text messaging as a tool for behavior change in disease prevention and management' was published in the peer reviewed journal, *Epidemiologic Reviews* (Cole-Lewis and Kershaw, 2010). This article was a systematic review of the peer-reviewed literature on behavior change interventions for disease management and prevention delivered through mobile text messaging through June 2009. As a requisite to be included in the review, the studies had to be randomized or quasi-experimental controlled trials of interventions that used text messaging as the primary mode of communication for disease prevention or management. Quality of study design was assessed using a standardized measure based on nine methodological characteristics and given a score of zero to 100 per cent.

Twelve studies met the inclusion criteria, with the earliest date of publication being 2005. The five disease prevention studies targeted preventive medication adherence, weight loss, physical activity, and smoking cessation. Of the seven disease management trials, only one targeted asthma management while the others focused on diabetes. The largest sample size was 1,705, but all other sample sizes ranged from sixteen to one hundred and twenty-six participants. The average age of participants in the study ranged from fifteen to forty-five years, with four studies specifically targeting adolescents and young adults. Intervention length ranged from three to twelve months, no studies had long-term follow-ups, and the frequency at which messages were sent varied greatly.

Only nine of the twelve studies included in the review were sufficiently powered to detect a difference in the intervention conditions. Of those nine, eight studies suggested that text messaging was a useful tool for behavior change. The utility of text messaging was supported for users of different ages, nationalities, and minority status. Only one of the nine countries represented in this study is considered a developing country. The review recorded characteristics of each intervention and attempted to identify gaps and issues in the literature, as well as best practices for researchers and practitioners. Issues identified include lack of scientific rigor, little representation of developing countries, and lack of use of behavioral theory.

Conducting the systematic review

The idea for this chapter was born out of my frustration as a public health doctoral student interested in the emerging field of mHealth in an environment where very few were yet engaged in it. Living in the academic research world, I found that whenever I would bring mHealth-related ideas into a discussion, my colleagues and professors would at least entertain my idea, perhaps even award the idea with the description of 'novel' or 'innovative', and then proceed with a litany of questions. They would rattle off the laundry list of common questions about the utility and feasibility of mHealth (for example cost of and access to mobile phones, level of general interest, issues of privacy and retention, and methods for evaluation). I would then reply to each of their points with facts about mobile phones and theories for why mHealth could be a catalyst to help solve many problems of the world. Regardless, no matter how many counterarguments I developed, or examples I provided of mHealth-related projects from websites of organizations with mHealth programs, there was one magic term my colleagues could always use to shut me down— 'evidence base'. I knew that once they asked for the evidence base, I would be stumped, because despite my conviction, I was also searching for evidence to substantiate the use of mHealth.

In my search to understand as much as possible about mHealth, I realized that there was a considerable amount of evidence in practice and gray literature, but I had trouble finding a true consensus in the peer-reviewed literature, which was sparse, at best. In the academic research world, novelty and innovation is encouraged. However, novelty and innovation with no evidence is shunned. I realized the strengths of mobile phones that made mHealth such a useful resource for healthcare and led to the rapid growth of their use in different practice settings (for example ubiquity, low cost, and relative ease of application with little need for infrastructure) were also the weaknesses that resulted in lack of formal documentation and application of systematic evaluation methodologies and ultimately a weak presence in the scientific peer-reviewed literature.

I felt that the little information that did exist required synthesis to allow people to understand the state of the literature, identify strengths and weaknesses, and thus better allocate resources. Through this, the evidence base for mHealth could be built upon, fostering growth, as opposed to everyone operating in their own respective silos and repeating the same projects only to come to the same conclusion, resulting in lateral instead of vertical growth. I observed the amount of money donors were putting into projects with the expectation of rapid results. I feared that the lack of a structured systematic approach to measuring outcomes would lead donors to lose interest and move on to the next novel idea with the assumption that mHealth does not work. Apart from my intuition, I knew there was something special in mHealth, as I bore witness to the way other industries (for example entertainment, marketing, and finance) were latching on to mobile technologies for their respective purposes. The vast majority of the industries using mobile technology are economically driven, which is a likely indication of effectiveness. Presumably, these profit-driven industries utilize mobile phones, because they are a cost-effective means of reaching their objectives.

Given my stance on mHealth, I realized that I was approaching the project with a potential bias. It was apparent that deep inside, I was rooting for mHealth. I realized the danger that this bias could pose to the scientific process, and therefore I became more determined to ensure that the methodology of the systematic review was scientifically sound. Furthermore, I braced myself with the reality that I could be completely wrong about mHealth, and in effect sought out to prove the opposite of what I believed (alternate hypothesis) – mHealth is not an effective tool for behavior change in disease prevention and management.

The paper was my small contribution to the vast amount of information available on mHealth. It is in no way exhaustive, but I hoped that it would give me some clarity and guidance as to what direction to move next. I specifically chose to focus on randomized controlled trials (RCTs) because they are typically considered the gold standard in scientific research. I am aware that much of the work that is being done in mHealth has not yet made it to the peer-reviewed literature, and that a majority of the work that does make it is not in the form of an RCT due to cost and methodological issues. Although I knew I would be missing some better-known projects, I also knew that the glaring omission of mHealth projects that people are most familiar with was just as powerful as including them in the paper.

I wanted to keep my methodology for the systematic review as rigorous as possible, and I knew the best way to do that was to streamline my ideas and focus on contributing something that had never been done before. I decided to limit the review to text messaging to highlight the utility of mHealth around the world for people of every socioeconomic status. Up to this point, I had found that when I explained mHealth to people, their first assumption was that mHealth could only be useful for people using iPhones or BlackBerrys, but given the successes that I had observed related to text messaging, I knew that this was not the case and wanted to make that point.

The decision to study disease prevention and disease management interventions separately came to me because each requires a different set of assumptions and actions. The motivators for engagement with an mHealth system will be different for someone who is actively managing a chronic condition as opposed to someone who is working to change a behavior to prevent the onset of a disease. In behavior change, we understand that the approach to behavior change differs depending on whether the condition of interest is primary, secondary, or tertiary. Therefore, we expected no difference when dealing with behavior change delivered via mHealth.

In order to ensure the most rigor for my review, I gathered resources that outlined the guidelines for literature reviews including the Cochrane Handbook for Systematic Reviews of Interventions, QUORUM guidelines, and the Handbook of Research Synthesis (Cooper and Hedges, 1994; Moher, Cook, Eastwood, Olkin, Rennie, and Stroup, 1999; Higgins and Green, 2009). I knew that I would need to tease apart the details of each intervention in order to correctly interpret the outcomes of a study. I had to understand exactly what type of service was delivered, how the service was delivered, and how the outcomes related to the service were measured. The Cochrane Handbook and similar resources allowed me to develop a systematic approach to the compilation of this data that would allow comparison between different interventions, while taking into account issues such as quality of study design.

In addition to general resources on how to conduct a rigorous literature review, I utilized other examples of literature reviews to better understand how to tailor the literature review guidelines to mHealth specifically. In this case, I did not limit myself to mHealth reviews. I also included reviews of interventions delivered via landline phones, the internet or computers through CD-ROM, as well as reviews of behavior change and health communication literature. Through these resources, I learned how to operationalize nuances specific to information communication technologies (ICTs). For instance, systematic review guidelines recommend a quality review of studies, since each study is not conducted with the same rigor; this should be taken into account when interpreting results. I soon realized that there were little to no published systems for quality review of mHealth interventions, but instead of creating a new one from scratch I was able to borrow and adapt an existing system from electronic health (eHealth) literature (Norman, Zabinski, Adams, Rosenberg, Yaroch, and Atienzan, 2007). This was an important lesson learned – while mHealth is relatively new, there remain many lessons to be drawn from other related bodies of literature. It is not always necessary to reinvent the wheel.

Once I dove into writing the paper, I came across a major limitation. I had originally set out to conduct a meta-analysis. This type of literature review would have allowed for the combination of data from each study in order to come to a statistical conclusion whether mHealth text messaging interventions were actually effective. Meta-analyses require that interventions be relatively homogenaous as far as outcomes measured, study designed, and methods employed. This was part of the reason I decided to define such narrow inclusion criteria for the reviews (i.e. only randomized controlled trials, only text messaging). However, the trials identified were still quite different. It soon became apparent that I would not be able to make any definitive statements on whether mHealth was more effective for one use or another (for example disease prevention versus management, young populations versus older populations).

At this point, I was unsure if the review would be worthwhile. After all, I was searching for definitive answers, and this limitation would make that impossible. I decided to push forward, in the hopes that the review could help others identify opportunities for research that would contribute to the literature and eventually provide enough data for future meta-analyses. In the end, I was happy that I did complete the review in the most systematic and rigorous way possible. Although the review did not provide the definitive answers I expected, feedback from those who read the paper after publication has led me to believe that the information provided in the review is valuable and may actually contribute to the vertical growth of the mHealth evidence base.

Lessons learned for mHealth research

The systematic review answered many questions, but it also unearthed more. The original question I sought out to answer was '*Does mHealth work?*'. However, with the advances of mHealth and contributions such as my systematic review, it is apparent that there are several more nuanced questions that must be addressed, such as '*How do mHealth interventions work?*', '*What particular aspect of an mHealth intervention is working?*', '*How much interaction with the mobile phone is necessary to observe a change in behavior?*', and '*What aspects of behavior are affected by mHealth and how?*'. Listed below are issues identified in the systematic review and lessons learned on how to address those issues:

Poor measurement as a result of no conceptual model for behavior change: In order to properly measure the impact of mHealth programs, we must first understand the pathways by which we expect to see change happen. It is important to remember that the health outcomes we expect to see are a result of a change in behavior, given interaction with a particular mHealth intervention. With no conceptualization of the proposed model of change, it can be difficult to determine what outcomes to measure. Practitioners can use logic models for intervention planning (i.e. inputs, outputs, short-term outcomes, and long-term impact). Systematic documentation of these aspects of the intervention as well as the behavior change strategy is important, and can strengthen the evidence base for mHealth, whether in the scientific or gray literature. Resources such as the United States National Cancer Institute's Pink Book – *Making Health Communications that Work* and the Johns Hopkins University Center for Communication Programs' *A Field Guide to Designing a Health Communication Strategy* provide practical guidelines for documentation of intervention strategies that can be helpful in the systematic design of formative research, as well as process and outcome evaluations (i.e. monitoring and evaluation systems) (O'Sullivan, Yonkler, Morgan, and Merritt, 2003; National Cancer Institute, 2011).

Lack of scientific rigor: There is a glaring need for more RCTs, as this is considered the gold standard for scientific evidence. RCTs can be expensive and are often not feasible for interventions conducted at the community level for various reasons. Where RCTs are not possible, creative options that utilize rigorous study design and analysis methods can be just as informative. Study designs such as the practical clinical trial (PCT), pragmatic randomized controlled trial (P-RCT), and the recently introduced cohort multiple randomized controlled trial (cmRCT) offer solutions to various limitations of RCTs such as issues of recruitment, ethics, as well as time and money constraints and provide data most relevant to decision makers (Hotopf, Churchill and Lewis, 1999; Hotopf, 2002; Tunis, Stryer and Clancy, 2003; Relton, Torgerson, O'Cathain, and Nicholl, 2010). More traditional alternatives such as repeated measures longitudinal study design or case-control design can also be informative. No matter what type of study design is employed, if the study is well documented and systematic, the lessons learned can be applied to many other situations. Furthermore, efforts should be taken to conduct power calculations prior to implementation of an intervention to ensure that the study will be able to detect a difference in the intervention groups. A robust study design is also imperative to conduct cost and cost-effectiveness analyses necessary to determine scalability and sustainability.

Lack of long-term follow-up: Studies included in this review did not conduct follow-up beyond the completion of the intervention. Interventions should attempt to conduct long-term follow-up in order to understand not only if the change in behavior was adopted, but also if the behavior was maintained. Furthermore, if measuring a health outcome that takes time to change, a longer follow-up period would allow investigators to determine if that change has actually occurred.

Little representation of developing countries in the scientific evidence: Randomized controlled trials in this review were conducted in nine countries, but only one was a developing country (Croatia) (Ostojic, Cvoriscec, Ostojic, Reznikoff, Stipic-Markovic, and Tudjman, 2005). This highlights the existing gap between the scientific literature and actual mHealth practice, as there are more mHealth interventions in developing countries documented in the gray literature (Mechael, Batavia, Kaonga, Searle, Kwan, Fu, and Ossman, 2010). There is a need for more systematic approaches to research and better scientific representation for work being conducted in low- and middle-income countries. This could be achieved through strategic partnerships and collaborations. Furthermore, it is useful to include regional databases when conducting literature searches. For instance, Literatura Latino-Americana e do Caribe em Ciências da Saúde (LILACS) is a database that indexes 670 health journals from the Latin American and Caribbean. An unbiased systematic review found that in one year, 71 percent of systematic reviews published in five high-impact medical journals could have been improved by including using LILACS to identify articles for inclusion in their analyses (Clark and Castro, 2002).

Inadequate intervention descriptions: There are many nuances that differ between programs such as whether information was tailored or not tailored, or delivered through one medium or multiple media, and whether messages were delivered a set number of times or based on the user's preference. These details are important to know when attempting to understand an intervention for the purposes of replication or comparison; however, seldom will descriptions from two different interventions report on all the same features of the program. Reasons for descriptive information not being included in the literature could be the result of a program not being systematic, or omissions considering space limitations of many scientific journals. Whatever the reason for the lack of details, the fact remains that the information is not available to practitioners and researchers who would like to critically interpret interventions for replication and comparison. Therefore, there is a need for a consensus as to what intervention description factors are most important, along with creative ways to measure and report on this information; even if it means sharing it with peer working groups, at conferences, on organization websites, or as electronic addenda for scientific journals. This sort of consensus would lead to the homogeneity necessary to conduct meta-analyses of the scientific literature that provide statistical conclusions on the effectiveness of specific types of mHealth interventions; a task that the systematic review discussed in this chapter was unable to complete, due to the heterogeneity of the literature.

Lack of behavioral theory use: The majority of the interventions in the systematic review failed to identify the use of a specific behavior change theory. Literature shows that use of a behavioral theory helps to make a program more successful. Therefore, the most apparent way to overcome this limitation is to design mHealth interventions using specific behavior change models, or at least a conceptual model using behavior change techniques. By contrast, the success of mHealth interventions despite lack of utilization of a formal behavior change theory leads to speculation, as noted in my systematic review, that there may be some unidentified aspects of behavior change theory that have been implicitly tapped by some mHealth interventions. While it is best to identify theory when the intervention is developed, there is information to be gained from those interventions with no explicit theory identified beforehand. Therefore, it may be useful to use qualitative methods to retrospectively explore interventions with seemingly little to no theoretical basis in order to determine if aspects of behavior change theory are in fact present. This is especially useful for those interventions that are developed rapidly in the field to address some specific need. Michie and colleagues have published guidelines that suggest using a formalized technique to determine if an intervention utilizes behavior change theory, and identify behavior change techniques that may not be specifically linked to an actual theory (Abraham and Michie, 2008; Michie, Johnston, Francis, Hareman, and Eccles, 2008; Michie and Prestwich, 2010). It is important to use a common taxonomy such as this when studying behavior change interventions, as it creates a common language and a metric system with which interventions may be compared. Retrospectively identifying theoretical concepts in existing interventions can also help practitioners to understand how to better include theory in their interventions. I suggest applying a mixed-methods approach to the evaluation of interventions: not only studying the typical quantitative questions such as the change in health outcomes, but also digging deep to understand the complexities of intervention components. Ultimately, whether through retrospective or prospective methods, we must determine what theoretical models are most successful for each situation, so that we may either replicate or move on to test another model.

Access to information: Even when mHealth-related information is published in the peer-reviewed literature, we run into an issue of access. The practitioners who may benefit from the information most and have immediate application for the evidence do not always have access to the articles because scientific journal subscriptions are often costly. This highlights the importance of publishing in open access journals and communicating with others engaged in mHealth through working groups and online communities. Often, when new information on mHealth is available, people will summarize relevant information and post for others to review and comment. Existing databases of mHealth-related content can be found through online communities such as the mHealth Toolkit, mobileactive.org, and the mHealth Alliance's HUB (K4Health, 2010; mHealth Alliance, 2010; MobileActive, 2010). People seeking access to these articles should also attempt to contact the corresponding author to request a complimentary copy of the research.

So where should we go from here?

Being trained as a behaviorist and epidemiologist, I am interested in closing gaps in the loop of mHealth knowledge by exploring the full model of behavior change. The purpose of mHealth research and evaluation is to identify the pathways by which mHealth interventions influence health outcomes. In other words, we seek to understand behavior change in the context of mHealth. Behavior change sits on the pathway between mHealth interventions and health outcomes. Technology utilization is also an important component of the model of change because it influences how much of the intended behavior change content a person experiences. It is important to identify how the characteristics of the mHealth technology, utilization of the technology, and effectiveness of the content shared through the technology influence the behaviors that lead to improved health outcomes.

In the context of mHealth, there is a continuum of behaviors of interest. First, there is the *health behavior* expected to be influenced through use of mHealth. The next is the person's *technology usage behavior*, referring to the way that the person engages or interacts with mHealth-related technology. Also of importance are the *mechanisms of behavior change* that the person is exposed to through interaction with the technology, which ultimately should lead to a *health behavior change.* The final result is a change in expected health outcomes, and ideally a *sustained healthy behavior*.

When evaluating the impact of an mHealth system, we cannot skip to measuring the health outcomes of the person, without understanding their technology use behavior. Similarly, we cannot skip from use of technology to measuring health outcomes, without understanding the mechanism of change by which we expect the health outcomes to improve. It is imperative to understand the overall model of change. For example, consider the following scenarios:

Scenario 1: Patient-level mHealth Intervention

Individuals receive a phone with a behavioral intervention to help self-manage their diabetes. We expect that each individual will interact with the phone and receive the behavior change content, which will encourage him or her to improve the targeted health behaviors, and eventually lead to improved health outcomes. *If the individuals do not have improvement in diabetes health outcomes, how do we know what part of the intervention does not work?* Did each individual utilize the features available on the phone in the same way and at the same frequency? Did the behavior change content provide the theoretical techniques necessary to influence behavior? Was this behavior change content appropriate to everyone utilizing the intervention, or should it have been tailored to address participants based on some predetermined characteristics? Was the user interface aesthetically pleasing? Were the health outcomes chosen for measurement the most appropriate, or are there intermediate psychosocial or behavioral characteristics that should have been monitored as well? Was the follow-up period long enough to observe the expected improvement in health outcomes?

Scenario 2: Provider-level mHealth intervention

Community health workers in rural villages receive mobile phones equipped with tools to improve efficiency of health delivery, and ultimately health outcomes. We expect the community health worker to make the behavior change necessary to incorporate the mobile phone into their work, which leads to the patient changing his or her behavior as instructed by the community health worker (take medication, visit health clinic, etc.). We expect these changes to lead to improved health outcomes for the entire village. *If we find that there is no change in health outcomes at the village level, how do we know what part of the intervention does not work?* Did each community healthcare worker use all the features of the mobile phone in the way we expected? How do we know that some community healthcare workers did not develop some new utility for the mobile phone which may have improved their personal workflow, but is different from the intended use? Did the patient adopt the behavior as expected? Was the model appropriate for the community health workers and/or the community? Were there some characteristics of the actual mobile phone intervention that made people more or less likely to interact with the technology? Was there adequate support in place to assist CHWs with the transition to incorporating the new technology in their existing workflow? Does the expected change in behavior actually lead to improved health outcomes? Was the follow-up period long enough to observe the expected improvement in health outcomes? Are there intermediate changes on the pathway to improved health outcomes that should have been considered?

Scenario 3: Population-level mHealth Intervention

A mass text messaging campaign is targeted toward a specific segment of the population to encourage them to adopt safe sexual practices. We expect that we send messages to a target audience, they are influenced by content of messages, they change behavior and this behavior leads to improved health outcomes at the population level. *If we find there is no change in health outcomes related to sexual practices, how do we know what part of the intervention does not work?* Did the messages actually reach the target population? Did the target population get the message but never read them? Did each member of target population read the same number of message? Did they all need the same number of message to initiate change? Did the content of the messages utilize the proper behavior

Table 3.1. Example scenarios and aspects of change model often missed during evaluation if pathways of change are not conceptualized beforehand.

Scenario	What we expect	What we normally measure	Technology Engagement (Dosage/ intended use vs. actual use)
1. Individuals receive a phone with a behavioral intervention to help manage diabetes care.	We expect that each individual will engage with the phone and receive the behavior change content, which will encourage them to change their health behaviors, and eventually lead to improved health outcomes.	Improved diabetes outcomes	Did each individual utilize the features available on the phone in the same way and at the same frequency?
2. Community health workers in rural villages receive mobile phones equipped with tools to improve efficiency of health delivery, and ultimately health outcomes.	We expect the community health worker to make the behavior change necessary to incorporate the mobile phone into his or her work, which leads the patient changing his or her behavior as instructed by the community health worker (take medication, visit health clinic, etc.), we expect these changes to lead to improved health outcomes for the entire village.	Village level health outcomes	Did each community healthcare worker use all the features of the mobile phone in the way we expected? How do we know that some community healthcare workers did not develop some new utility for the mobile phone which may have improved their personal workflow, but is different from the intended use?

What we may miss (Other possible measures)			
Mechanism of Change (Behavior Change Theory)	**Appropriateness of Intervention Design**	**Outcomes Measured**	**Length of Follow-up**
Did the behavior change content provide the theoretical techniques necessary to influence behavior?	Was this behavior change content appropriate to ever yone utilizing the intervention, or should it have been tailored to address participants based on some predetermined characteristics? Was the user interface aesthetically pleasing?	Were the health outcomes chosen for measurement the most appropriate, or are there intermediate psychosocial or behavioral characteristics that should have been monitored as well?	Was the follow up period long enough to observe the expected improvement in health outcomes?
Did the patient adopt the behavior as expected?	Was model appropriate for the CHWs and/or the community? Was there some characteristics of the actual mobile phone intervention that made people more or less likely to interact with the technology? Was there adequate support in place to assist CHWs with the transition to incorporating the new technology in their existing work flow?	Does the expected change in behavior actually lead to improved health outcomes? Are there intermediate changes on the pathway to improved health outcomes that should have been considered?	Was the follow up period long enough to observe the expected improvement in health outcomes?

Continued

Table 3.1. Continued

Scenario	What we expect	What we normally measure	Technology Engagement (Dosage/ intended use vs. actual use)
3. A mass text messaging campaign is targeted towards a specific segment of the population to encourage them to adopt safe sexual practices.	We expect that we send messages to a target audience, they are influenced by content of messages, they change behavior, and this behavior leads to improved health outcomes on the population level.	Health outcomes of the target population related to sexual practices	Did the messages actually reach the target population? Did the target population get the messages but never read them? Did each member of target population read the same number of message? Did they all need the same number of message to initiate change?

change theories or techniques most effective with this population? Was this mode of delivery appropriate for the target population? Are there some participants who would have benefitted better from an actual downloadable application? Would some have preferred messages delivered more or less frequently? Were messages the appropriate length? Does this behavior actually lead to the expected health outcome? Was the follow-up time long enough to recognize a change in health outcomes? Were there some intermediate outcome measures that could indicate that health outcomes would eventually improve?

Taking advantage of technology utilization information to form usage metrics can help form the intermediate variables needed in order to measure mediators and moderators of the expected outcome, and answer many of the questions identified by the scenarios presented in the text and in Table 3.1. MHealth and other ICTs allow unique opportunities for analysis because so much information is captured that is not available in traditional behavior change interventions. There are many opportunities to utilize data that is not traditionally collected for the purposes of research.

What we may miss (Other possible measures)			
Mechanism of Change (Behavior Change Theory)	**Appropriateness of Intervention Design**	**Outcomes Measured**	**Length of Follow-up**
Did the content of the messages utilize the proper behavior change theories or techniques most effective with this population?	Was this mode of delivery appropriate for the target population? Are there some who would have benefitted better from an actual downloadable application? Would some have preferred messages delivered more or less frequently? Were messages the appropriate length?	Does this behavior actually lead to the expected health outcome? Were there some intermediate outcome measures that could indicate that health outcomes would eventually improve?	Was the follow-up time long enough to recognize a change in health outcomes?

For example, in the case of the mHealth intervention mentioned in Scenario 2, data collected for the purpose of improved service delivery could also be utilized to create aggregate reports for epidemiologic surveillance (Table 3.1). With creativity, we are able to utilize data that ordinarily would not be considered research worthy. For instance, in Scenario 1 system usage metrics such as how long or how often a person accessed a particular feature of the mHealth intervention would allow you to understand how much that person used the system and develop metrics that allow the measurement of what aspects of the intervention are most likely to bring about change (Table 3.1).

As observed in my systematic review, interaction within many mHealth programs is voluntary, meaning participants can decide what aspect of the intervention to utilize and at what frequency. The result is that different people will use it in different ways. In effect, people begin to self-tailor because they use the parts that are most convenient or relevant to them. For example, in Scenario 3, one user may only pay attention to text messages that offer interactive questions with the opportunity to respond, while another may only read text messages that provide knowledge and suggest an action for overcoming a related barrier (Table 3.1). It can be viewed as an organic tailoring process. It is therefore important for us to parse out the details of this usage behavior to determine how and why different types of users utilize different aspects of an intervention, and if it ultimately leads to change.

Conclusion

In order to understand why an mHealth intervention does or does not have an impact, we must first conceptualize the mechanisms by which we expect change to happen for each specific aspect of the intervention. Using an overall model of change during the design, implementation, and evaluation stages of an mHealth intervention can prevent throwing the proverbial baby out with the bath water; meaning that when an intervention does not reach expected outcomes, instead of dismissing it as an unsuccessful intervention altogether, researchers are able to tease apart the various aspects of the intervention to determine where the breakdown in the expected model of change occurred and also ensure that the proper intermediate outcomes are being measured.

For example, Ritterband and colleagues have suggested an overall model of behavior change for internet interventions that can also be applied to mHealth interventions. The model proposes that behavior change occurs through nine nonlinear steps (Ritterband, Thorndike, Cox, Kovatchev, and Gonder-Frederick, 2009). Each person approaches the intervention with a certain set of *user characteristics* that influence their *website use*. Website use is also influenced by *website characteristics* and *support*. Engagement with the website leads to *behavior change*, *symptom improvement*, and *treatment maintenance* through various *mechanisms of change*. Every step of the model can be influenced by *environmental* factors (Ritterband *et al.* 2009). While this model is specific to internet interventions, it is applicable to mHealth interventions and underscores the importance of drawing from the related fields of eHealth and other ICTs for social change initiatives.

There is an ecosystem of health that already exists; the overlay of mobile phones has only made this ecosystem more fluid and is allowing it to progress rapidly. Each mHealth intervention will take a different approach depending on circumstances and the resources available. At the end of the day, no one project will answer all the questions of mHealth, but if we are able to make strategic partnerships, build upon lessons learned from other ICT-related research, develop sound and systematic documentation of methods, and apply rigor in evaluations, we will eventually be able to piece it all together. In the future, there will be more information available to create a comprehensive picture of where each project stands in the mHealth ecosystem and allow us to move forward swiftly and bring about change.

References

Abraham, C. and Michie, S. (2008), 'A Taxonomy of Behavior Change Techniques Used in Interventions', *Health Psychology* 27(3): 379–87.

Clark, O. and Castro, A. (2002), 'Searching the Literatura Latino-Americana E Do Caribe Em Ciencias Da Saude (LILACS) Database Improves Systematic Reviews', *International Journal of Epidemiology* 32: 112–4.

Cole-Lewis, H. and Kershaw, T. (2010), 'Text Messaging as a Tool for Behavior Change in Disease Prevention and Management', *Epidemiologic Reviews* 32(1): 56–69.

Cooper, H. and Hedges, L. (1994), *The Handbook of Research Synthesis*, New York: Russell Sage Foundation Publications.

Higgins, J. and Green, S. (2009), 'Cochrane Handbook for Systematic Reviews of Interventions: Version 5.0.2', *The Cochrane Collaboration*, http://www.cochrane-handbook.org [Accessed 25 October 2009].

Hotopf, M. (2002), 'The Pragmatic Randomised Controlled Trial', *Advanced Psychiatric Treatment* 8: 326–33.

Hotopf, M., Churchill, R. and Lewis, G. (1999), 'Pragmatic Randomised Controlled Trials in Psychiatry', *British Journal of Psychiatry* 175: 217–23.

K4Health. (2010), 'mHealth Toolkit', http://www.k4health.org/toolkits/mhealth [Accessed 15 February 2012].

Mechael, P., Batavia, H., Kaonga, N., Searle, S., Kwan, A., Fu, L. and Ossman, J. (2010), Barriers and Gaps Affecting mHealth in Low and Middle Income Countries: Policy White Paper. New York, Center for Global Health and Economic Development, Earth Institute, Columbia University.

mHealth Alliance. (2010), 'Hub: Health Unbound', http://www.mhealthalliance.org/hub [Accessed 15 February 2012].

Michie, S., Johnston, M., Francis, J., Hardeman, W. and Eccles, M. (2008), 'From Theory to Intervention: Mapping Theoretically Derived Behavioural Determinants to Behaviour Change Techniques', *Applied Psychology* 57(4): 660–80.

Michie, S. and Prestwich, A. (2010), 'Are Interventions Theory-Based? Development of a Theory Coding Scheme', *Health Psychology* 29(1): 1–8.

MobileActive. (2010), 'Mobileactive.Org: A Global Network of People Using Mobile Technology for Social Impact', http://www.mobileactive.org [Accessed 10 December].

Moher, D., Cook, D., Eastwood, S., Olkin, I., Rennie, D. and Stroup, D. (1999), 'Improving the Quality of Reports of Meta-Analysis of Randomized Controlled Trials: The Quorom Statement. Quality of Reporting of Meta-Analyses', *Lancet* 354(9193): 1896–900.

National Cancer Institute (2011), 'Pink Book 2011: Making Health Communication Programs Work', Washington, DC: http://www.cancer.gov/pinkbook [Accessed 15 February 2012].

Norman, G., Zabinski, M., Adams, M., Rosenberg, D., Yaroch, A. and Atienzan, A. (2007), 'A Review of Ehealth Interventions for Physical Activity and Dietary Behavior Change', *American Journal of Preventive Medicine* 33(4): 336–45.

O'Sullivan, G., Yonkler, J., Morgan, W. and Merritt, A. (2003), *A Field Guide to Designing a Health Communication Strategy*. Baltimore, Johns Hopkins Bloomberg School of Public Health/Center for Communications Programs.

Ostojic, V., Cvoriscec, B., Ostojic, S., Reznikoff, D., Stipic-Markovic, A. and Tudjman, Z. (2005), 'Improving Asthma Control through Telemedicine: A Study of Short Message Service', *Telemedicine Journal and eHealth* 11(1): 28–35.

Relton, C., Torgerson, D., O'Cathain, A. and Nicholl, J. (2010), 'Rethinking Pragmatic Randomized Controlled Trials: Introducing the "Cohort Multiple Randomised Controlled Trial" Design', *BMJ* 340: 963–7.

Ritterband, L., Thorndike, F., Cox, D., Kovatchev, B. and Gonder-Frederick, L. (2009), 'A Behavior Change Model for Internet Interventions', *Annals of Behavioral Medicine* 38(1): 18-27.

Tunis, S., Stryer, D. and Clancy, C. (2003), 'Practical Clinical Trials: Increasing the Value of Clinical Research for Decision Making in Clinical and Health Policy', *JAMA* 290(12): 1624–32.

4 Developing and Adapting a Text Messaging Intervention for Smoking Cessation from New Zealand for the United Kingdom

Caroline Free, London School of Hygiene and Tropical Medicine, University of London

Background

Tobacco use is a leading cause of preventable death, estimated to cause more than five million deaths each year worldwide (WHO, 2009). Around half of current smokers will be killed by their habit if they continue to smoke and 25 percent to 40 percent of smokers will die in middle age (Doll, Peto, Boreham, and Sutherland, 2004; Vollset, Tverdal and Gjessing, 2006). In the US and the UK over half of existing smokers report they would like to stop (Lader, 2009; McClave, Whitney, Thorne, Mariolis, Dube, and Engstrom, 2010).

Existing effective behavior change smoking cessation support interventions include group, one-on-one, and telephone counseling. These increase smoking cessation by pooled relative risk of 1.98, a 95 percent confidence interval of 1.60 to 2.46 for group counseling, pooled relative risk of 1.39, a 95 percent confidence interval of 1.24 to 1.57 for individual counseling, and pooled relative risk of 1.29, a 95 percent confidence interval of 1.20 to 1.38 for telephone advice (Lancaster and Stead, 2005a; Stead, Perera and Lancaster, 2006; ITU, 2010). However, many smokers cannot or do not want to use existing services. Additional effective interventions to support smoking cessation are urgently needed.

Mobile phone technology has the potential to provide personalized smoking cessation support. Motivational messages and behavior change tools used in face-to-face smoking cessation support can be modified for delivery via mobile phones with the content tailored to the age, sex, and ethnic group of the quitter (Rodgers, Corbett, Bramley, Riddell, Wills, Lin, and Jones, 2005; Free, Whittaker, Knight, Abramsky, Rodgers, and Roberts, 2009). In this way, support can be delivered wherever the person is located, without them having to attend services and can be interactive, allowing quitters to obtain extra help when needed (Rodgers *et al.*, 2005; Free *et al.*, 2009).

Because of the widespread ownership of mobile phones, fully automated smoking cessation support can be delivered to large numbers of people at low cost. In 2009, more than two thirds of the world's population owned a mobile phone and 4.2 trillion text messages were sent (ITU, 2010). In the UK, there are about 120 mobile phone subscriptions per 100 population with ownership greater than 80 percent in all socio-economic groups (Ofcom, 2009).

The STOMP (Stop smoking with mobile phones) trial, conducted among 1,700 young smokers (at least sixteen years of age with a mean age of twenty-five years) throughout New Zealand, assessed the effectiveness of a text message-based smoking cessation intervention (Rodgers *et al.*, 2005). The STOMP intervention text message content was developed by a motivational interviewing trained counselor, Tim Corbett, and contains over 1,000 text messages. The trial results showed considerable promise, with over a twofold increase in self-reported quit rates at six weeks (28 per cent versus 13 per cent, relative risk 2.2, a 95 per cent confidence interval of 1.79 to 2.70, p-value of less than 0.0001). The results were consistent and separately significant across all major subgroups including those defined by age, sex, ethnicity, income level, and geographical location. Some limitations in the study, however, affected the validity of the results at six months. First, there was differential loss to follow-up at six months (79 per cent follow-up in the control group versus 69 per cent in the intervention group). This is likely to be due to the control group receiving a month of free text messaging in return for continuing to participate until the 26-week follow-up call, while the intervention group was not offered this. Second, only a small sample of self-reporting quitters was selected for biochemical validation through salivary cotinine testing.

The txt2stop intervention in the UK was modified and developed from the STOMP intervention and was evaluated in a randomized controlled trial with 5,800 participants (Free, Cairns, Whittaker, and Edwards, 2008; Free *et al.*, 2009). The txt2stop intervention is a complex intervention, as it contains a number of components providing information combined with a range of behavior change techniques. Participants are asked to set a quit date within fourteen days of randomization. There is frequent contact by text message (five messages per day) in the first five weeks after randomization and then messages reduce to three per week for six months. Specific features of the intervention include that: participants can opt to have a 'quit buddy' where participants with similar characteristics and quit dates are paired up so that they can text each other for support. Participants can also text the word 'crave' or 'lapse' at any time, and a text message (or series of text messages) is immediately delivered in response.

Existing guidance for the development and evaluation of complex interventions suggests that the key elements of the process include development, feasibility and piloting, evaluation, and implementation phases (Craig, Dieppe, Macintyre, Michie, Nazareth, and Petticrew, 2008). The developmental phase includes identifying an evidence base for the intervention and identifying or developing appropriate theory and modeling process and outcomes. Feasibility and piloting can involve testing procedures, estimating recruitment and retention, and determining sample sizes. Evaluation can involve evaluating effectiveness, understanding change processes, and assessing cost-effectiveness (Craig *et al.*, 2008).

I will report the work we completed in chronological order from the work completed prior to the txt2stop pilot trial through to the main trial.

Development

The work we completed prior to the main trial was twofold, first to modify the existing STOMP intervention for a UK population and second to generate new messages.

Modifying the existing text messages

To modify the existing content of the STOMP text message intervention for the UK, the STOMP messages were first reviewed by smoking cessation counselors employed by the QUIT smoking cessation charity working in the UK. Their views regarding the comprehensibility, suitability, and content of messages were sought. Suggestions for improvements in messages were incorporated and texts were modified. All text messages were subsequently assessed in a series of focus groups by sixty-two potential trial participants (smokers, ex-smokers, and smokers trying to quit).

All text messages were reviewed in at least two focus groups to assess their acceptability, comprehensibility, and participants' response to the messages (did they find them encouraging/discouraging, would they like to receive such messages, and would such messages help or hinder them if they were trying to quit). Where text messages were 'liked' in both groups they were retained. If a text message was 'disliked' by any member of either group, further questions were asked to explore what was 'disliked'. Participants and smoking cessation counselors were asked for their suggestions in improving the messages. Any messages that were altered were subsequently tested in at least two further focus groups. The process was repeated until the message was considered comprehensible and acceptable in at least two groups. Where messages were not rendered acceptable and comprehensible they were discarded.

Feedback from the focus groups was extremely positive regarding both the concept of txt2stop and the text message content. Four main types of modification were made: changes to words, for example reflecting different terms or text abbreviations used in the UK, changes to culturally specific references, for example to music and sports personalities, changes to the framing of text messages, for example to involve more 'suggestion' and less 'telling', and changes or removal of some texts, such as texts which participants found 'too American' or 'patronizing'. Changes to framing and removal of some messages were completed based not only on participants' feedback but also on the theoretical basis of our approach to generating new smoking cessation messages described later in the chapter.

Generating new messages

Existing guidance for the development of complex intervention suggests that intervention development be informed by theory and the existing evidence base (Craig *et al.*, 2008); however, it remains unclear which theories would result in the most effective interventions. While the existing evidence base shows that group, individual, and telephone counseling are effective in increasing smoking cessation, there was no clear evidence demonstrating which components of these interventions are most important or necessary to increase smoking cessation (Stead, Lancaster and Perera, 2003a; Lancaster and Stead, 2005a; Stead and Lancaster, 2005a). Thus in the absence of clear evidence regarding which theory should be used, we examined and drew on a range of theories to develop the txt2stop intervention. These included psychological behavioral theories and behavior change techniques and approaches, social theory (and contextual data), and theories regarding therapeutic relationships (doctor–patient relationships). As there was no clear evidence about which elements of face-to-face smoking cessation counseling are most effective, we worked with practicing smoking cessation counselors modifying the approaches they used for delivery by text message. We describe how each theory and our work with smoking cessation counselors generated specific types of messages.

Psychological theories of health behavior and behavior change

There are a wide range of psychological theories of health behavior and health behavior change. These include social cognition models (such as the theory of planned behavior), as well as dynamic theories of behavior changing (such as stages of change and spontaneous processing models). In addition, the discipline of psychology provides a wide array of techniques and approaches used in psychological interventions to change behavior (such as the techniques use in motivational interviewing).

Social cognition models

Social cognition models aim to describe the factors influencing behavior. The theory of planned behavior (Ajzen, 1985), for example, suggests that the proximal determinants of behavior are the intentions to engage in the behavior and perceptions of control over the behavior. Intentions represent a person's motivation in the sense of her or his conscious plan or decision to exert effort to perform the behavior. Intention is determined by three sets of factors: beliefs about the behavior, which is a product of beliefs about outcomes and the evaluation of the outcome. Secondly, subjective norms are the person's belief about whether significant others think he or she should engage in the behavior, which is function of normative beliefs. This is operationalized as 'does the individual's referent think the person should perform the behavior' and the motivation to comply with the referents expectation. The third determinant is perceived behavioral control, which is the perception of ease or difficulty of the behavior. Judgments of perceived behavioral control are influenced by beliefs concerning whether one has access to the necessary opportunities and resources to perform the behavior successfully. This includes internal control factors, information, personal deficiencies, skills, abilities, emotions, and external control factors such as opportunities, dependence on others, and barriers.

While such theories may inform our understanding of behavior in isolation, social cognitive psychological theories of behavior (such as the theory of planned behavior) were too removed from the specific beliefs and motivations influencing smoking to directly inform the content of messages. Such theories could lead researchers to generate text messages aiming to influence beliefs about outcomes such as the health benefits of the behavior they are promoting but require contextual data which may be socially or culturally specific to inform researchers regarding smokers' beliefs and motivations regarding their behavior. A further limitation of such models in informing which messages should be developed is that such theories are theories of behavior not theories of behavior change. Thus while the importance of motivation for example is emphasized, the theories do not tell you how to increase motivation. As such, they describe the factors influencing behavior but do not necessarily provide a clear mechanism for influencing these factors or the behavior itself. Social cognition theories are based on subjective expected utility theory and deliberative reasoning processes (for example weighing up the pros and cons of behavior). The limitations of such approaches in understanding behavior have been outlined; for example, Fishbein and Fazio have described the importance of the salience and accessibility of attitudes (Fishbein and Ajzen, 1975; Fazio, 1990). A further limitation of such theories is that they are static and do not take into account changes over time.

Dynamic theories of behavior

Dynamic theories of behavior acknowledge that both motivation and behavior vary at different times and some theories acknowledge that changes may occur over short time periods in the same individual. The stages of change model (Prochaska and DiClimente, 1984) describe smokers going through precontemplation (not even thinking about quitting) and contemplation phases (thinking about quitting) prior to being ready to quit and then maintaining quitting or relapsing. However, this theory was of limited use for informing the content of our intervention, as eligibility criterion for the trial was that all participants were willing to make a quit attempt in the next month and were currently daily smokers. Thus our intervention was not designed for smokers at precontemplation or contemplation phases described by the stages of change model, but specifically only included smokers ready to attempt a change.

Salience of attitudes and spontaneous processing models

Fishbein and others focus on the salience of attitudes in informing behavior (Fishbein and Ajzen, 1975). Fishbein claims that any person may possess a large number of beliefs but that at any one time only some of these are likely to be salient. It is the salient beliefs that determine attitude to the behavior and behavior. This view is supported by evidence from cognitive psychology which suggests that people have poor information processing ability and therefore are unlikely to consider all their beliefs. With this modification of decision making, it becomes important to identify beliefs salient to the individual.

Fazio goes further in his theory of 'spontaneous processing models' (Fazio, 1990). He argues that people only make decisions weighing up the pros and cons of a behavior when they have both the opportunity and motivation to do so. He states that social cognitive variables will predict behavior according to these models when these conditions are met. In this theory, not all social behavior is deliberative or reasoned but is more spontaneous in nature. Thus he describes two means of decision making. The first is conscious decision making in which an individual analyzes the costs and benefits of a particular behavior and deliberately reflects on the attitudes relevant to the behavioral decision. The second means of decision making is a spontaneous reaction to one's perception of the immediate situation. In such a model, the individual may not have actively considered the relevant attitudes and/or not be aware of the influence of attitude. The attitudes may influence how the person interprets the event that is occurring. An attitude will be automatically triggered from memory following the presentation of relevant cues. The likelihood of activation is determined by the accessibility of the attitudes, which in turn is a function of how strongly the attitude is linked to the behavior and how the person evaluates the attitude. Once activated the attitude shapes the perception in an automatic attitude congruent fashion, i.e. if a positive attitude is activated this leads person to notice positive qualities of the attitude object. This automatic process of selective perception will therefore shape the individual's definition of the event and thus determine behavior. Furthermore, recent activation or priming of an attitude from memory is sufficient for that attitude to influence interpretations and priming can be subliminal (the individual need not consciously reflect on the attitude).

According to spontaneous processing models, participant's perceptions and hence response to a situation depend on whether the individual's attitudes are activated from memory. The situation provides cues but the key to behavior is the attitude accessibility.

Experimental work, conducted outside the health arena, supports key aspects of these theories namely that accessibility of relevant attitudes influences the strength of relationship between attitudes and behavior and that highly accessible attitudes can lead to selective perception (Fazio, 1990).

In relation to text message-based smoking cessation support, Fazio's spontaneous processing models and theories regarding the importance of salience of attitudes a text messaging smoking cessation intervention might provide insight into how the messages could work (Fazio, 1990). One potential advantage of text messaging interventions lies in their ability to reach participants wherever they are at any time, as mobile phones are generally always carried by participants (Rodgers *et al.*, 2005; Free *et al.*, 2009). In txt2stop, text messages are sent at intervals throughout the day and every day. Text messages could act to prime positive attitudes relating to quitting that are held by the smoker so that such attitudes are stronger and more accessible when cues for smoking occur. Thus the text messages sustain the salience and accessibility of quitting attitudes and motivations over smoking attitudes and motivations. So, when stimuli to smoking occur, it is the smokers' quitting attitudes that are retrieved from memory rather than their smoking attitudes.

A further potential advantage of text messaging interventions is that unlike face-to-face, telephone, or internet interventions where the participant has to have sufficient motivation to seek help and support, in text message-based interventions messages can be delivered which have not been specifically sought at that time. Thus messages could provide affirmation regarding the quit attempt, remind participant why they are quitting, and boost motivation to continue with the quit attempt at times when motivation for quitting is low or waning. These theories, relating to the potential mechanism of action of text messages, did not directly inform the precise content of messages. Based on these theories, it was important for messages to be positive, target smokers reasons for quitting and staying quit, boost motivation and be delivered at intervals throughout waking hours (for example *Quitting smoking is the most important thing you can do to improve your health. Quit for you and protect those around you*).

Those generating messages were made aware of these practical implications of the theory, but were not necessarily aware of the psychological theory underpinning these requirements.

Techniques and approaches used in existing behavior change interventions

To develop text messages using behavior change techniques and approaches found in existing smoking cessation interventions, we also drew on the ethos and techniques used in motivational interviewing and the approaches used by existing telephone and face-to-face smoking cessation counselors. Many of such techniques and approaches are routed in therapeutic psychology. Motivational interviewing uses a range of techniques face-to-face (Miller and Rollnick, 2002). Motivational interviewing is client-centered and the emphasis is on exploring the participant's motivations, choices, and empowerment. Some of the techniques used in motivational interviewing include exploring ambivalence about behavior change, decisional balance (pros and cons), reflective listening, resisting telling participants what they should do, understanding patient motivations, listening with empathy, and empowering participants to achieve their own objectives using open questions and summarizing. The automated txt2stop intervention was not capable of responding to individual motivations and responses in the way an MI counselor can in a one-on-one session. We did, however, incorporate some elements of motivational interviewing into the programmer. The STOMP and txt2stop interventions text messages asked participants about the pros and cons of quitting for them (decisional balance), for example *TXT2STOP: If u think quitting is v important, you're more likely to stay quit. List pros and cons of smoking.* Some messages asked participants their reasons for quitting (which many participants responded to by text message), for example *TXT2STOP: Why not write an action list of your reasons why you want to Quit. Use it as your inspiration.* In the pilot work, elements of text messages that were directive and telling participants what they should do were removed and replaced with options (choices). Messages were sent which affirmed both the decision to quit and provided congratulations regarding having quit (after the quit day), such as *Well done, 2 wks quit, don't weaken now, uv gone thru the worst – don't allow yrslf to get addicted again!*

Messages showed empathy to participants for example acknowledging that quitting was hard but encouraging them to keep going, for example *Don't be too hard on yourself. Quitting smoking can make you feel angry or sad at things that normally would not bother you.*

As existing evidence demonstrates that face-to-face and telephone counseling is effective in supporting quitting, we also drew on the knowledge and experience of trained smoking cessation counselors (Stead, Lancaster and Perera, 2003b; Lancaster and Stead, 2005b; Stead and Lancaster, 2005b). Smoking cessation counselors use a range of behavior change techniques, and experienced counselors can have expertise in the best ways of framing support and the kind of language that smokers respond to and understand. To date, it remains unclear which techniques are essential or more effective in supporting quitting, so smoking cessation counselors were asked to generate messages based on their experience (Stead *et al.*, 2003b; Lancaster and Stead, 2005b; Stead and Lancaster, 2005b). We included text messages covering any approach smoking cessation counselors described using that we could feasibly deliver by text message, given the restrictions imposed on us by the text messaging technology which had limited interactivity and personalization and only 160 characters for each text message. Smoking cessation counselors provide support and encourage smokers to used medications, so additional text messages were developed to encourage participants to use nicotine replacement therapy in addition to the txt2stop support. Some messages were developed based on theories that we generated with the counselors. For example, counselors commented that many smokers liked the information they gave about the benefits to smoker's body and health that would achieve by stopping smoking. We hypothesized that the ability to send text messages at specific times co-inciding with the time that the benefit would occur would be particularly motivating. For example, oxygen levels become normal eight hours after stopping smoking. The program was set up to send the following message to participant hours after stopping. *TXT2STOP: Health update! Well done, your oxygen levels are now normal. Check out your web page www.txt2stop.org to see how you're getting healthier.*

Contextual evidence

Contextual evidence regarding smokers' beliefs and motivations can be obtained from qualitative and cross-sectional quantitative research. Much of this research is routed in social theory, which emphasizes the sociocultural influences on behavior. Clearly, our text message-based intervention was directed to individual smokers, although it included interpersonal support, thus its ability to address broader social influences on behavior is extremely limited. However, qualitative research and cross-sectional surveys rely on data from individual smokers and provide considerable and detailed understanding of the beliefs, social norms, and motivations that influence behavior. We provide one example of how we used such data. The QUIT smoking cessation charity had completed focus groups exploring smokers' beliefs regarding nicotine replacement therapy (NRT); smokers reported that they did not use NRT as they were concerned nicotine was as harmful as cigarettes. They had limited awareness of the other chemicals present in cigarette smoke that cause harm. For the pilot trial, we therefore developed text messages addressing these misconceptions, for example *TXT2STOP: Nicotine makes you want another cigarette but it's the 4,000 other chemicals in smoke that can kill you. Nicotine replacement therapy helps you quit* and *You will be twice as successful if you quit smoking and use an NRT product.*

Theory regarding doctor–patient relationships and interactions

In models of doctor–patient relationships and consultations engaging the patient and establishing rapport is the first step in a consultation (Pendleton, Scofield, Tate, and Havelock, 1984; Neighbour, 1987). In clinical settings, engaging the patient and establishing rapport is carried out through a number of techniques including the use of open-body language and taking a 'patient-centered' approach. Establishing 'engagement and rapport' in an automated text message intervention represented a particular challenge. All nonverbal cues are absent, and body language could not be used to make participants feel welcome to the program. In addition, the program has limited interactive content limiting its ability to adopt an individual approach. Thus, language and messages that were designed to be welcoming and developing a sense that the people behind the text messages were real people who were concerned about the smoker. *TXT2STOP: Don't try to quit smoking on an exam day or if you have a job interview – try to quit on a day that is stress free.* Or *TXT2STOP: If you have any questions about TXT2STOP, you can contact the team free from a landline call to 0800 xxxxxxxx.* (The research team if contacted were able to answer questions about the trial and did not offer smoking cessation advice). While it was not possible to fully individualize the intervention, both STOMP and txt2stop interventions were able to address issues that arise with smokers trying to quit such as concerns about weight gain and concerns about friends smoking.

Fine tuning new messages

Generating messages which were only 160 characters long was a particular challenge. Short messages mean that the most important element of the message had to be determined to fit into one text message or the messages had to be split into two components sent in separate messages at different times. In addition,

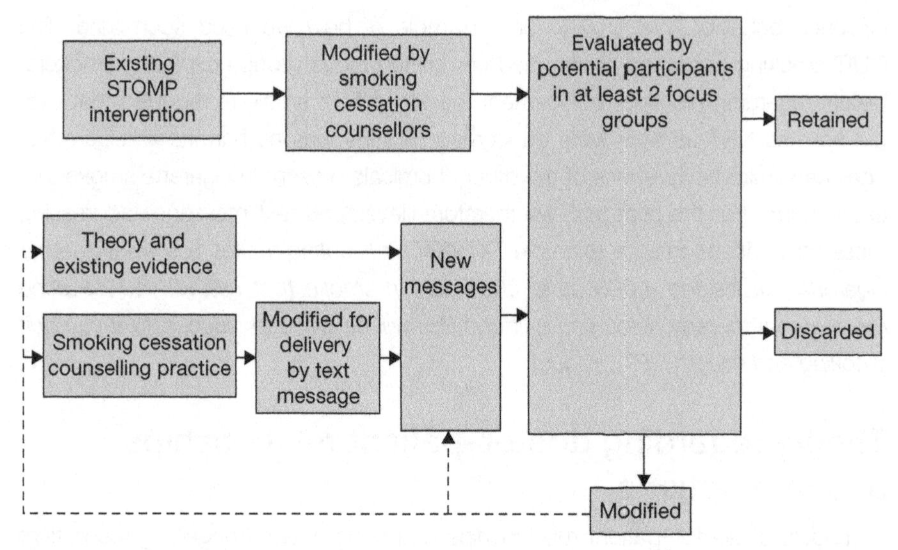

Figure 4.1 The process used to generate text messages for the txt2stop intervention

messages had to be framed and using language that was acceptable to people. Other challenges are related to the limitations of an automated program in responding to individuals. We used the same methodology to fine tune the content of new messages as we used to modify the messages in the existing STOMP program. All new messages were tested in at least two focus groups to assess their acceptability, comprehensibility, and participants' response to the messages. Messages were modified until at least two focus groups found them acceptable and comprehensible, or the messages were discarded (Figure 4.1).

Feasibility and piloting

The feasibility of delivering the txt2stop intervention and trial methods was assessed in a pilot trial with 200 participants. A full account of the pilot trial is reported elsewhere (Free *et al.*, 2009).

The pilot randomized controlled trial aimed to recruit and recruited successfully 200 participants. We recruited the target of 200 participants within seventeen days from the trial launch and had to close the trial to further recruitment. Our computer-based data collection and randomization systems worked efficiently, as did the interfaces between the web-based data collection system, the computer program generating texts, and the SMS company which sent the text messages to the participants. All text messages sent were received by the trial participants.

Using evidence-based methods for follow up, we achieved 98 percent complete short-term follow-up and 92 percent long-term follow-up. The short-term results showed a doubling of self-reported quitting relative risk of 2.02, a 95 percent confidence interval of 1.08 to 3.76, and the effects at six months were consistent with a modest benefit in the point prevalence of biochemically validated smoking cessation with a relative risk of 1.28 and a 95 percent confidence interval of 0.46 to 3.53 (8.5 percent or 8/94 versus 6.7 percent or 6/90).

The process evaluation for the pilot trial

The qualitative statements made by the participants in the intervention group showed that participants value the intervention, for example '*It's a good effort from u guys thanks for stopping me*' and '*thank you very much for allowing me on the program and for helping me quit I'm sure my daughters would thank you if they understood*'. The text messages were described as '*very good*', '*incredibly helpful*' and '*very motivating*'. In particular, participants' comments illustrate the quality of communication that can occur through text messages: '*I found myself talking myself out of having another cigarette when my buddy was the one craving one. I think this process helped even if it was reverse psychology*'. Some participants' comments illustrate how unique components of the intervention can help quitting: '*text crave was a good function especially when out*' or '*Every time I was craving a cigarette I'd get a text and it would stop me. They'd always arrive at the right time*'. Quit buddies were described as '*great*' and '*brilliant*'. Participants also suggested modifications to the program. Three participants wanted to reset their quit date. Three participants were disappointed with their quit buddy, who did not respond to their text messages. Others wanted to set their own start time for the messages. A number of participants commented that they did not want to receive messages in using texting abbreviations and several participants asked for more messages regarding the health benefits of quitting.

Process evaluation questionnaires were completed by 56 percent (n = 57/102) of the participants in the intervention group. Of these, 96 percent (n = 54) reported that the text messages in plain English were easy to understand and 61 percent (n = 34) thought the messages in text lingo were easy to understand. Fifty-six percent (n = 31) reported that it was useful being able to embargo times and 27 percent (n = 15) wanted to be able to embargo an additional time. The number of text messages received was: about right for 44 percent (n = 25) respondents, too few for 14 percent (n = 8) respondents, 5 percent (n = 3) were unsure and 37 percent (n = 21) of respondents thought it was too many. Nineteen percent (n = 11) liked using the text crave function and 21 percent (n = 12) liked having a 'QUIT buddy'. Sixty-eight percent (n = 39) would recommend the txt2stop program to a friend, 21 percent (n = 12) would not and 11 percent (n = 6) were unsure if they would recommend the program to a friend. Thirty-one percent (n = 17) of the participants who completed a process evaluation questionnaire reported that they had successfully quit at six weeks. Sixty percent (n = 34) reported that the text messages using 'standard English' were useful in helping them quit, 34 percent (n = 19) reported that the text lingo messages were useful in helping them quit, 30 percent (n = 12) thought having a 'QUIT buddy' was useful in helping them quit and 32 percent (n = 8) reported that the text CRAVE option was useful in helping them quit.

Development

Based on the findings from the pilot trial and process evaluation, a number of changes and additions were made to the txt2stop intervention. The intervention was modified, so trial participants were able to reset their quit date, had greater flexibility regarding embargoing times that they did not want to receive messages, and could choose the start time for messages. Participants could opt to change their quit buddy. Additional messages regarding the health benefits of quitting were added. The pilot trial results demonstrated that many participants relapsed between four weeks and six months following their quit date, so further work focused on the development of messages to strengthen the intervention in supporting participants to cope with cravings and to avoid relapse. The existing evidence base regarding relapse prevention provides limited evidence regarding effective interventions (Hajek, Stead, West, Jarvis, and Lancaster, 2009). We therefore interviewed smoking cessation counselors regarding the steps they took in support people who lapsed and in trying to prevent relapse. Based on this messages were developed focusing on planning for dealing with cravings and temptation to smoke (for example *TXT2STOP: To make things easier for yourself, try having some distractions ready for cravings, and think up some personal strategies to help in stressful situations*). In addition, a new feature was added to the program where participants who had smoked a cigarette were advised to text LAPSE to the short code. In response, participants would receive a series of three messages in succession designed to reassure the participant that this did not need to be the end of their quit attempt, encourage the participants to think about why they had lapsed and make a plan of how to prevent this in the future and encourage them to restart their quit attempt, such as *T2S: Don't be too hard on yourself. If you've slipped, you haven't failed. Quitting is a process. You've managed to stop for a while and that's an incredible achievement. Keep going!*

Evaluation

The main trial conducted with 5,800 participants showed that the intervention more than doubled biochemically verified smoking cessation at six months (Free, Knight,

Robertson, Whittaker, Edwards, Zhou, Rodgers, Cairns, Kenward, and Roberts, 2011). In addition to the main trial, we conducted qualitative interviews with twenty-five participants and completed a process evaluation with 600 participants. Participants were also asked to provide feedback regarding the messages. Full account of the methods and results of these evaluations will be published elsewhere. Here, I will describe the key findings from the quantitative process evaluation and discuss the extent to which they support or refute the benefits of particular messages or the theories underpinning the messages.

In the process evaluation, a twenty-two item questionnaire was used and statistical significance was set at a p value of 0.002 using a bonferoni adjustment. Participants in the intervention group were statistically significantly more likely to report that they saved messages on their phone to re-read, that they were aware craving would get easier over time, and that the messages encouraged them to stay quit when I felt like smoking. In the intervention group 15 percent (n = 25) and in the control group 6 percent (n = 11) of participants reported 'yes' to the statement '*the text messages made me want to smoke*'.

The quantitative evidence from the process evaluations suggests that from participants' perspectives, the role of the messages in supporting motivation to stay quit is important. Participants in the intervention were more likely to be aware that cravings would get easier over time and to have written a list down of their reasons for quitting, but the process evaluation cannot tell us if these factors were causal in increasing quitting or the product of another causal pathway such as engagement in the intervention. Being aware that cravings get easier over time could also be an outcome of successful quitting. In feedback, participants also stated that messages about the benefits that their body and health were obtaining from quitting were especially motivating.

The findings from the process evaluation are consistent with the hypothesis that the intervention works predominantly by maintaining the salience and accessibility of 'quitting/ staying quit' attitudes to sustain motivation and quitting over time. The messages also appeared to prompt smoking in some participants, which suggests that the messages can increase the salience and accessibility of quitting or smoking attitudes and potentially cue behavior in opposing ways. Participant accounts are also in keeping with our theory that receiving messages regarding the benefits that their body was experiencing at the time this occurred after quitting was especially motivating.

Further work should explore the factors that influence the level of support experienced by participants and participants' experience of the interventions as a 'real person'. Further work is needed to identify why participants respond in different ways to the messages and which participants experience cravings for smoking on receipt of messages. Following the development of the intervention, we coded the text message content using a typology of behavior change techniques (Michie, Free and West, submitted for publication). In the future, work developing new text messaging interventions could be informed by recent research describing behavior change techniques and their effectiveness, which was not published when we developed the txt2stop intervention (Michie, Hyder, Walia, and West, 2011; Michie, van Stralen and West, 2011). Future work on text messaging interventions for smoking cessation support should explore ways of improving the txt2stop intervention, potentially involving the use of a greater range of behavioral techniques, further tailoring of the intervention and fine-tuning the intervention based on participants' feedback.

Summary

The work we completed followed key processes outlined in existing guidance for the development and evaluation of complex interventions. We worked on theory, the existing evidence base, and the existing STOMP program to generate text messages, which were evaluated and modified using feedback from smoking cessation counselors and potential participants in focus groups. The messages were subsequently tested in a pilot trial. Feasibility of the trial process (recruitment, follow up) and delivery of the intervention were assessed in the pilot trial. Findings from the process evaluation for the pilot trial were used to further develop the intervention. The intervention was subsequently evaluated in a main trial. Thus we moved forward and backward between development, piloting, and evaluation phases to finalize the txt2stop intervention evaluated in the main trial. Plans for implementation have been initiated. A similar methodology could be used to develop other texting messaging interventions.

References

Ajzen, I. (1985), 'From Intentions to Actions: A Theory of Planned Behaviour', in J. Kuhl and J. Beckmann (eds), *Action Control: From Cognition to Behaviour*, Heidelberg: Springer: 11–39.

Craig, P., Dieppe, P., Macintyre, S., Michie, S., Nazareth, I., and Petticrew, M. (2008), 'Developing and Evaluating Complex Interventions: The New Medical Research Council Guidance', *BMJ* 337: a1655.

Doll, R., Peto, R., Boreham, J. and Sutherland, I. (2004), 'Mortality in Relation to Smoking: 50 Years' Observations on Male British Doctors', *BMJ* 328(7455): 1519.

Fazio, R. (1990), 'Multiple Processes by Which Attitudes Guide Behavior: The Mode Model as an Integrate Framework', *Advances in Experimental Social Psychology* 23: 75–109.

Fishbein M and Ajzen I (1975), *Belief, Attitude, Intention and Behaviour:An Introduction to Theory and Research*, Reading MA: Addison-Wesley.

Free, C., Knight, R., Rodgers, A., Whittaker, R., Cairns, J., Edwards, P., Roberts, I., Txt2stop: a randomised trial of cell-phone text-messaging to support smoking cessation in the UK. *The Lancet Protocol Reviews* (2008).

Free, C., Knight, R., Robertson, S., Whittaker, R., Edwards, P., Zhou, W., Rodgers, A., Cairns, J., Kenward, M., Roberts, I., Smoking cessation support delivered via mobile phone text messaging (txt2stop): a single-blind, randomised trial Lancet 2011:378;49-55.

Free, C., Whittaker, R., Knight, R., Abramsky, T., Rodgers, A. and Roberts, I. (2009), 'Txt2stop: A Pilot Randomised Controlled Trial of Mobile Phone-Based Smoking Cessation Support', *Tobacco Control* 18(2): 88–91.

Hajek, P., Stead, L., West, R., Jarvis, M. and Lancaster, T. (2009), 'Relapse Prevention Interventions for Smoking Cessation', *Cochrane Database of Systematic Reviews* 2009(1): CD003999.

ITU. (2010), 'The World in 2010 ICT Facts and Figures', www.itu.int/ITU-D/ict/material/FactsFigures2010.pdf [Accessed 15 February 2012].

Lader, D. (2009), Opinions Survey Report No. 40. Smoking-Related Behaviour and Attitudes, 2008/09. Newport, Office for National Statistics.

Lancaster, T. and Stead, L. (2005a), 'Individual Behavioural Counselling for Smoking Cessation', *Cochrane Database of Systematic Reviews* 2005(2): CD001292.

Lancaster, T. and Stead, L.F. (2005b), 'Individual Behavioural Counselling for Smoking Cessation', *Cochrane Database Syst Rev*(2): CD001292.

McClave, A., Whitney, N., Thorne, S., Mariolis, P., Dube, S. and Engstrom, M. (2010), 'Adult Tobacco Survey: 19 States, 2003–2007', *Morbidity and Mortality Weekly Report: Surveillance Summaries* 59(3): 1–75.

Michie, S., Free, C. and West, R. (submitted for publication), 'Characterising the "Txt2stop" Smoking Cessation Text Messaging Intervention in Terms of Behaviour Change Techniques', *submitted for publication*.

Michie, S., Hyder, N., Walia, A. and West, R. (2011), 'Development of a Taxonomy of Behaviour Change Techniques Used in Individual Behavioural Support for Smoking Cessation', *Addictive Behavior* 36(4): 315–9.

Michie, S., van Stralen, M. and West, R. (2011), 'The Behaviour Change Wheel: A New Method for Characterising and Designing Behaviour Change Interventions', *Implementation Science* 6.

Miller, W. and Rollnick, S. (2002), *Motivational Interviewing: Preparing People for Change*, New York: Guilford Press.

Neighbour, R. (1987), *The Inner Consultation*, Lancaster: Kluwer Academic Publishers.

Ofcom (2009), 'The Consumer Experience: Telecoms, Internet and Digital Broadcasting 2009. Evaluation Report', London: Ofcom. http://stakeholders.ofcom.org.uk/market-data-research/market-data/consumer-experience-reports/eval09/ [Accessed 15 February 2012].

Pendleton, D., Scofield, T., Tate, P. and Havelock, P. (1984), *The Consultation: An Approach to Learning and Teaching*, Oxford: Oxford University Press.

Prochaska, J. and DiClimente, C. (1984), *The Transtheoretical Approach: Crossing Traditional Boundaries of Therapy*, Homewood: Dow Jones Irwin.

Rodgers, A., Corbett, T., Bramley, D., Riddell, T., Wills, M., Lin, R. and Jones, M. (2005), 'Do U Smoke after Txt? Results of a Randomised Trial of Smoking Cessation Using Mobile Phone Text Messaging', *Tobacco Control* 14(4): 255–61.

Stead, L. and Lancaster, T. (2005a), 'Group Behaviour Therapy Programmes for Smoking Cessation', *Cochrane Database of Systematic Reviews* 2005(2): CD001007.

Stead, L., Lancaster, T. and Perera, R. (2003a), 'Telephone Counselling for Smoking Cessation', *Cochrane Database of Systematic Reviews* 2003(1): CD002850.

Stead, L.F., Lancaster, T. and Perera, R. (2003b), 'Telephone Counselling for Smoking Cessation', *Cochrane Database Syst Rev*(1): CD002850.

Stead, L., Perera, R. and Lancaster, T. (2006), 'Telephone Counselling for Smoking Cessation', *Cochrane Database of Systematic Reviews* 3: CD002850.

Stead, L.F. and Lancaster, T. (2005b), 'Group Behaviour Therapy Programmes for Smoking Cessation', *Cochrane Database Syst Rev*(2): CD001007.

Vollset, S., Tverdal, A. and Gjessing, H. (2006), 'Smoking and Deaths between 40 and 70 Years of Age in Women and Men', *Annals of Internal Medicine* 144(6): 381–9.

WHO (2009), WHO Report on the Global Tobacco Epidemic, WHO. Geneva, WHO.

5 mHealth Hope or Hype

Experiences from Cell-Life

Peter Benjamin, Cell-Life

Introduction

We are a social species – since humanity first evolved we have wanted to communicate within our family, community, clan, and more recently within our nation and globally. To communicate with everyone has been a dream in many cultures (for example, the Tower of Babel) and the ancient Greeks believed only the gods could express themselves so all could hear (it was called the weather).

In the last century, our species learned how to do rapid mass communication with radio, TV, and mass-circulation newspapers. In the last couple of years for the first time we have mass interaction. Today, in countries like South Africa, where 90 per cent of youths and adults have a cellphone (World Wide Worx, 2010), almost anyone just about anywhere can communicate with nearly anyone else, immediately and at a low cost (relative to any other way of doing this). This is extraordinary; it has the potential to transform how society is organized. We are just starting to explore what this means – many clever people have learned how to make lots of money. How can this be used to promote people making better choices around their health (part of what is known as Behavior Change Communications)? Well, I am not sure yet; and this is the story of the first steps of Cell-Life exploring what is possible with this new technology.

Cell-Life beginnings

Cell-Life is a not-for-profit company (Section 21 in SA law) based in Cape Town, South Africa, which develops open-source computer systems to support the health and HIV sector. This chapter describes the evolution of Cell-Life over a decade, and then gives some reflections on the hope and hype of mHealth.

Cell-Life started as a research project at the University of Cape Town in 2000 when two academics, Professor Jon Tapson and Dr Ulrike Rivett, decided to explore ways that electrical engineering could be used for social good. They were soon joined by Dr Jevon Davies of the Cape Peninsula University of Technology.

The first project in 2001 was a simple system for home-based carers (who support around a dozen AIDS patients each) to report back to the clinic on the patients' conditions. This system worked quite well at the Hannan Crusaid Clinic in Gugulethu (a township around Cape Town) run by the Desmond Tutu HIV Foundation (DTHF), the HIV clinical research center in Cape Town. However, the team learned that not only engineering factors matter. After the first week of the project, when the carers (who were all women) were asked how it was going, they said that they did not like cellphones. The Cell-Life team had bought good quality phones with the right technical specification, so they were surprised to hear this. In 2001, cellphones were not common, and the carers felt nervous carrying the big cellphones on the street and in public transport. After a discussion, they asked for cellphones small enough to hide in their bras. This was something the mainly male Cell-Life engineers had not considered.

After receiving funding from the Vodacom Foundation and others, in 2004 Cell-Life set up as a separate nonprofit organization. Cell-Life's second main product was a database system to assist pharmacists in dispensing anti-retroviral drugs (ARVs). The DTHF was one of the first organizations to provide ARVs which they dispensed from their main office at Groote Schuur Hospital which were delivered to township clinics for the patients to pick up. It was difficult to keep track of who received which drugs, therefore the request to develop a system for tracking the medicine. This became the 'Intelligent Dispensing of Anti-Retroviral Therapy' (iDART) system, which was installed first in clinics in the Western Cape, then in North-West province, then nationally. In this process, we started learning the complexities of working inside the health system – this was before there was comprehensive ARV access, and there was a great deal of politics around the HIV program. While pharmacists tended to like the system as it simplified their work, it was difficult to get people higher-up in management structures to make decisions. It took us several years to work the best way to engage with the health system, which was made much easier when we employed a medical doctor, Dr Sikki Noor Mohammed, who knew how the system worked and who to talk to.

Cellphones for HIV

I joined Cell-Life in 2007. Since 1990 I had been working in what became known as 'Community Informatics', the use of information and communication technology (ICT) for community development. First, this was in my home country, the UK, with Poptel, GreenNet, and the Manchester Host (a municipal email and bulletin board system in the early 1990s). In 1994, I moved to South Africa and worked in several organizations trying to use ICTs to support the social change in the newly liberated

South Africa. My PhD studied the efforts to establish telecentres. My thesis was largely a catalogue of the many technical, organizational, and financial ways these community ICT projects failed. It was very difficult keeping a center with a few PCs working in dusty remote areas with poor electricity, a community where very few people knew how to use computers and there was inadequate money to keep the equipment functioning. The people who benefitted were the few who learned computer literacy, and then left to get jobs in the cities. What we thought were local development projects in practice led to the best and brightest leaving the area (though they often sent money home to their families).

I was a slow learner. It took me about a decade to notice that about half the people in the village around the telecenter already had a cellphone, which compared with a PC had much better connectivity, worked more easily, people were much more comfortable to use and was accessible in a way that the telecenter would never be.

As I started to see the potential that cellphones could have, the job as general manager of Cell-Life became available. In my first few months, I asked of my contacts in the ICT and telecommunications field '*Who was doing HIV communications?*', and all the people I was meeting in the AIDS sector '*Who was using cellphones to communicate?*'. To my increasing surprise, I learned that no one was. This was confirmed for me at the National AIDS Conference in June 2007 when I spent two days walking around the fifty stands in the exhibition hall asking all the organizations if they were using mobile tech in their communications: they were not, though half of the organizations expressed interest.

With some funding support from Vodacom and also the RAITH Foundation, we started the 'Cellphones for HIV' (C4H) project in 2007 as an attempt to introduce the HIV sector in South Africa to the use of mobile technology as a means of communicating within organizations and between organizations and their constituency. A first stage in the project was to develop the technical systems and gain operational experience. This took longer than we hoped – about a year and a half. While the techies were building an SMS engine we called 'Mobilisr' (together with a partner organization, the Praekelt Foundation), during 2008 we became a part of the wider HIV sector, learning the communications and clinical needs of the myriad of organizations, and as we were the first group talking about mobile communications and HIV, we were offered a seat on the Communications Task Team of the South Africa National AIDS Council (SANAC), which was a great place to understand the sector.

By 2010 our technology capacity included: SMS (broadcast out, and IN with keywords); USSD (basic text menus that all GSM cellphone can use that allows simple information retrieval and data collection); MXit (a massively popular cellphone instant messaging system used by over 20 million people in South Africa, especially youths, and we provided the HIV content on this); Location Based Services (knowing where a cellphone is for '*Where is my nearest something?*' services); Please-Call-Me (a means for someone with no 'airtime' to ask a colleague to phone them back – which is the only free way to send a signal from a cellphone which we use for people to subscribe to services at no cost) and Cellbooks for downloading large volumes of text to a cellphone.

These technologies were used in various ways, to meet the needs of our different partners. Cell-Life was learning how to apply the tools to meet health and social objectives. The tools were used to support different areas of HIV and health communications, including:

1. Mass communication for prevention with over 2.5 million SMSs sent to around 300,000 people;
2. Information for positive living (via SMS, USSD, and MXit);
3. Linking patients and clinics (adherence and appointment reminders, mainly using SMS);
4. Text counseling (we linked MXit with the National AIDS Helpline, so people could have 'text-counseling', and there have been over 21,000 counseling conversations since September 2009);
5. Organizational capacity building (providing subsidized or free SMS and USSD services to over 100 government, NGO, and community HIV organizations);
6. Monitoring and evaluation.

mHealth grows up

I was lucky enough to attend the Rockefeller Foundation Conference in Bellagio in August 2008 that started to crystallize the field of mHealth. It was exciting to learn from many others and feel that a new field was coming together (Atun and Sittampalam, 2006; Kaplan, 2006). After that workshop, we started seeing much of our work using mobiles in the HIV sector as part of mHealth.

In the last few years, there have been several other organizations in South Africa involved in mHealth projects, including GeoMed, the Centre for Scientific and Industrial Research, the Medical Research Council, Praekelt Foundation, Stellenbosch University, Right To Care, and the Reproductive Health Research Unit (RHRU). Most of the projects were fairly small scale, with all of us trying to find evidence to convince the government or a donor of the importance of mHealth.

However, the environment changed dramatically in mid-2010 when the National Department of Health received 15,000 good quality cellphones as part of the Universal Service Obligations of cellphone companies. During 2011, the rollout of two cellphones to all 4,300 public health facilities would begin. After a decade of largely failing to get an internet computer in each facility (today only around 1,500 of the 4,300 facilities have a working email address), in the next few months there should be the first comprehensive health informatics network throughout all facilities. The first thing the Department of Health want to do with this is to have a cellphone-based reporting system of HIV counseling and testing (it was a high priority to test 15 million people for HIV in 2011). After a tender procedure, Cell-Life, with our partner the Health Information Systems Program, received the contract to implement this in late 2010. This is definitely bigger than other projects we have done before – training 14,000 people at around 7,000 public and private health facilities. I am confident we will be able to deliver, but nervous to realize the new scale we are working at. Be careful what you ask for – you just might get it!

There is currently great attention around mHealth, almost a feeding frenzy. The mHealth Summit in Washington, DC in November 2010 showed the wide range of organizations involved in this new area with 2,500 people and dozens of organizations and projects (Mechael, 2009; Vital Wave Consulting, 2009; Cole-Lewis and Kershaw, 2010; Mechael, Batavia, Kaonga, Searle, Kwan, Fu, and Ossman, 2010). In particular, data collection systems, SMS messaging, and smartphone apps were everywhere. However, there was very little evidence. There were a handful of projects that actually could prove medical benefit through randomized controlled trials or similar; almost nothing that had gone to scale – Text4Baby (Centers for Disease Control and Prevention, 2010) and the TRACnet clinical reporting in Rwanda (Svoronos, Jilson and Nsabimana, 2008) being about the only examples – and absolutely no examples of a clear business case or serious health economic cost-benefit analysis. MHealth as a field is just emerging. Probably there will only be two or three years of such attention: the many overhyped ideas will fade away, while the really useful applications will not be called mHealth – it will simply be the obvious way to perform a particular task (just as there is not a Stethoscope Society – everyone can see it is the appropriate tool and so uses it).

Great – so what?

Did any of this have any effect? Just counting SMSs is not evaluation. At the organizational level, many organizations working in healthcare and HIV are now using mobile technology. On the World AIDS Day on December 1, 2008, and 2009,

SANAC asked us to use many mobile tools (broadcast SMS, location-based services to find local events, the MXit-text counseling, and USSD menus for information), and they now consider cellphones as a channel for all communications such as TV, radio, and newspapers. To get a better assessment of the impact of these tools, we have run some formal studies (funded by Right To Care) into various applications.

One study tested whether SMS support messages can improve the outcomes of prevention of mother-to-child transmission of HIV (PMTCT). This was a randomized trial at a maternity hospital in Johannesburg (Coronationville Hospital) with 386 HIV+ mothers who (after informed consent) received SMSs for ten weeks after birth on various topics: Reminders to give babies HIV-prevention medication; encouragement on exclusive feeding; appointment reminders; new motherhood tips, and other positive living messages for those who were newly diagnosed with HIV. The study finished around August 2011, and preliminary results so far show a significant increase in the percentage of mothers who take their babies for testing at six weeks (58 per cent of those not receiving bring their babies in comparison to 74 per cent of those receiving SMSs; $p<0.001$). But proper data will only be available on publication. Surveys of those who received SMSs indicate that they are appreciated and are seen as supportive and informative. Some mothers indicated that the SMSs helped them to accept their HIV status.

In another study called 'SMS to Test', we examined whether a series of SMSs giving information and encouraging people to take HIV tests would result in their testing. The SMSs dealt with common barriers to testing (as identified in the literature), and provided referral for where to get help with these issues. We also had two kinds of messaging: 'informational' content with HIV statistics and public health announcements; and 'motivational', which talked about taking control of one's life and respecting loved ones. Over 2,500 people were enrolled, and divided into groups: group one received no SMSs (the control), group two received three SMSs with 'informational' content, group three received ten informational SMSs, group four received three 'motivational' SMSs, and the last group, group five, got ten motivational SMSs. After the SMS campaign, recipients were surveyed to see whether they had tested for HIV, and whether the SMSs had affected their decision to test. The only intervention that showed an increased rate of HIV testing was the ten motivational messages.

We have also set up a system for HIV 'text-counseling'. Since August 2009, Cell-Life has worked with LifeLine, the NGO that runs the well-respected National AIDS HelpLine or NAHL (Katz, 2004). We have built a technical link between MXit and the NAHL so that people can have text conversations with professional counselors on any HIV issue. Counselors were trained to provide counseling via a web-based Instant Messaging application. By January 2011, around 24,000 conversations had happened and we are assessing its effectiveness. Users are surprisingly revealing things such as their HIV status and sexual behaviors. It is also clear that people still need basic information on HIV (like whether it is transmitted by kissing, or the fact that with medication you can live a long life). Anecdotal evidence from the counselors indicates that they can provide as much meaningful counseling in one two-hour session as they can in a week of telephone counseling. One reason for this is that they can have multiple conversations at the same time, and they have many fewer hoax calls. They have also indicated that mobile-chat counseling affords the client a degree of privacy not possible with telephone counseling: with the latter the counselors often hear background traffic noise (from public telephones) and clients using 'bland' language (not mentioning HIV), whereas on mobiles, clients can text-chat from anywhere with greater privacy. Cost is a major factor in the popularity of the service and its potential for scale-up and rollout in other countries. A counseling conversation using mobile voice costs the user US$1 in the region (for a four-minute call); a similar conversation on MXit costs less than US$0.01. This provides a means for organizations to provide low-cost call center services via text counseling.

To date, Cell-Life has run various cellphone-based systems that seem to be liked by the users, but we are just beginning to be able to show any direct medical benefits.

What's different about mobile?

What is unique to mobile about these applications? Over nearly ten years, Cell-Life has learned to use mobile communications in different ways. Our first projects were around data collection for healthcare workers, and then we started providing services to patients. We have explored using the tools in different ways – from simple information reminders (for example adherence reminders), to emotionally supportive messaging seeking behavior change (for example the SMS to Test study), to two-way interaction (such as the National AIDS Helpline text counseling).

We have learned that as well as simple information, mobile technology can provide significant emotional support (Mefalopulos, 2008). The SMSs sent in the PMTCT mentioned above were valued: when asked why she would recommend the SMS, one woman said, '*Because it feels like whatever heavy you carried on your shoulders, that it actually becomes and feels much lighter.*' When asked whether the SMSs made the women feel better, various responses were, '*It made me believe that all will be ok*', '*It gave me strength, I just felt better since I know that I am not alone and that you people also care about us and you know what we are going through*', and '*Having a new baby is very stressful but by getting these*

SMSs it always made me excited.' Compared with most health infrastructure of buildings, equipment, and trained staff, cellphone messaging is a cheap and easy intervention – yet it can have a real impact. A mobile phone is a very intimate medium – people usually keep it on their person, and it can be a very useful tool to support people through difficult times.

Mobile allows interaction to support other forms of communication (such as TV, radio, print, and mobile) where messages from other media are extended via mobile, or where interactivity via mobile is added to traditionally 'one-way' campaigns. This is one of the areas in which cellphones can greatly strengthen health communications – allowing people to 'talk back' to broadcast media. Behavior change communication is most effective when there is a dialogue rather than simply a one-way flow of information. However, broadcast media are very poor at allowing interaction – radio phone-ins or letters to the editor do not provide a meaningful one-on-one conversation. Cellphones can be used to allow people to interact with the TV or radio communications (Winchester III, 2009). For example, after a program on a given topic, viewers can be encouraged to SMS in their comments; vote in a poll; join a subscription list by sending an SMS (or Please Call Me) to a number; or find their local clinic or health facility by an SMS/Please Call Me to another number. If they want to discuss the issue, they can go to an Instant Messaging chat room (such as through MXit); or if they have a serious issue they can seek counseling. This can allow the wide reach of the broadcast medium to be the first stage of an ongoing interaction.

Mobile also allows narrowcasting, where a message is targeted at the small population to whom the message should be relevant. If the demographics or interests of people are known, then mobile phones provide an easy way to reach this population (as would an email if they have the facility, or a normal letter if there is the time). For me, the big news is not that this technology is mobile. The main issue is that almost everyone has one – cellphones are nearly ubiquitous in countries like South Africa.

If you do not have medical aid, live in a rural area, and are feeling unwell, you have three choices. Firstly, you could do nothing and hope it gets better (which is actually what happens in most cases). Secondly, you could go to the public clinic (either an hour's walk or expense of bus/taxi) with all the inconvenience of travel, childcare, time off work (if employed). There, you wait for a few hours to then get five minutes of attention from a hassled, overworked nurse who *may* diagnose you correctly, and possibly has the appropriate medication and then there is the long trip home. This has taken most of a tiring day (and remember, you are already feeling sick). The third choice is to go to a traditional healer, who probably lives close to your house, will probably be nice to you, and will listen properly to what you have to say. The human interaction between a caregiver and patient is therapeutic itself and at the heart of curative medicine. By some estimates, there are ten times more traditional healers than registered health professionals in the country. This is usually discussed in terms of traditional versus educated world views; but it also is a measure of how inaccessible the conventional health system is to the majority of people in these contexts. There is a possibility of using mobiles to increase access to scientific healthcare through near-universal access to primary health information, access to triage counseling to give an indication of whether you need to go to the clinic, and widespread promotion of preventative health.

As Clay Shirky has said, 'These tools don't get socially interesting until they get technologically boring' (Shirky, 2009). It is not the few thousand iPhones in South Africa that will make a major difference – but if we can find a way to turn these electronic-connected devices in the pockets of 90 per cent of youths and adults into means of accessing a range of medical services that could transform healthcare. However, while cellphones provide a means of reaching a very large number of people, it must be remembered that there are a significant number of people who do not have access to this technology. Health communications that assume universal cellphone usage will leave out the people who are likely to be the most disadvantaged – which can lead to a form of 'double exclusion'.

Different from other forms of telemedicine or electronic health (eHealth), mHealth can talk about aspects of healthcare beyond just the curative (fixing people when they know they are ill). Because a majority of people can use these tools regularly in their lives (and not only when visiting a clinic), mobile tools can build health awareness, enhance preventative healthcare, and support well-being and overall wellness. This is a much wider agenda for technology in healthcare than ICT and medicine usually covers.

Cell-Life is currently working on ways to provide useful health applications through basic phones – 'smart apps for dumb phones'. These health applications could range from basic lifestyle services (such as losing weight, stopping smoking, doing exercise, and eating well), through general health information (for example health services, primary healthcare info), condition-specific services (such as adherence to medication, self-managed care for TB, diabetes, and hypertension), and health administration (booking appointments, receiving updates), to medical consultations and counseling.

We have just started to learn how to use this new technology. As cellphones are in the hands of the great majority, mobile technology provides an opportunity to increase equity in the provision of quality health services. There is a huge amount of work to do.

References

Atun, R. and Sittampalam, S. (2006), 'A Review of the Characteristics and Benefits of SMS in Delivering Healthcare', in Vodafone (ed), *The Role of Mobile Phones in Increasing Accessibility and Efficiency in Healthcare*, London: Vodafone. http://www.vodafone.com/etc/medialib/public_policy_series.Par.38545.File.dat/public_policy_series_4.pdf [Accessed 15 February 2012].

Centers for Disease Control and Prevention. (2010), 'Text4baby for Pregnant Women and New Moms', http://www.cdc.gov/Features/Text4Baby/ [Accessed 15 February 2012].

Cole-Lewis, H. and Kershaw, T. (2010), 'Text Messaging as a Tool for Behavior Change in Disease Prevention and Management', *Epidemiologic Reviews* 32(1): 56-69.

Kaplan, W. (2006), 'Can the Ubiquitous Power of Mobile Phones Be Used to Improve Health Outcomes in Developing Countries?', *Globalization and Health* 2: 9.

Katz, I. (2004), 'The South African National AIDS Helpline: Call Trends from 2000–2003', http://www.cadre.org.za/node/170 [Accessed 8 March].

Mechael, P. (2009), 'The Case for mHealth in Developing Countries', *Innovations: Technology, Governance, Globalization* 4(1).

Mechael, P., Batavia, H., Kaonga, N., Searle, S., Kwan, A., Fu, L. and Ossman, J. (2010), Barriers and Gaps Affecting mHealth in Low and Middle Income Countries: Policy White Paper. New York, Center for Global Health and Economic Development, Earth Institute, Columbia University.

Mefalopulos, P. (2008), 'Development Communication Sourcebook: Broadening the Boundaries of Communication', http://web.worldbank.org/WBSITE/EXTERNAL/TOPICS/EXTDEVCOMMENG/0,,contentMDK:21890561~pagePK:34000187~piPK:34000160~theSitePK:423815,00.html [Accessed 24 May].

Shirky, C. (2009), 'Clay Shirky: How Social Media Can Make History', http://www.ted.com/talks/clay_shirky_how_cellphones_twitter_facebook_can_make_history.html [Accessed 20 February 2012].

Svoronos, T., Jilson, I. and Nsabimana, M. (2008), 'Tracnet's Absorption into the Rwandan HIV/AIDS Response', *International Journal of Healthcare Technology and Management* 9(5): 430–45.

Vital Wave Consulting (2009), mHealth for Development: The Opportunity of Mobile Technology for Healthcare in the Developing World. Washington, DC & Berkshire, UN Foundation - Vodafone Foundation Partnership.

Winchester III, W. (2009), 'Catalyzing a Perfect Storm: Mobile Phone-Based HIV-Prevention Behavioral Interventions', *interactions* 16(6).

World Wide Worx. (2010), 'Mobile Internet in South Africa 2010', http://www.worldwideworx.com/archives/250. [Accessed 4 June 2010].

6 Tele-Self-Management Support for Type 2 Diabetes Care

Working through public primary care centers in Santiago, Chile

Ilta Lange, WHO/PAHO Collaborating Center for Primary Health Care, Pontificia Universidad Católica de Chile

Introduction

Type 2 diabetes is a chronic disease and a cardiovascular risk factor of high physical, psycho-social, and economic impact. Like many countries, Chile is experiencing a dramatic increase in rates of diabetes as well as of diabetes risk factors, such as obesity and a sedentary lifestyle. Its prevalence is 9.4 per cent and much higher among people with lower socio-economic status and minimal formal education (Ministerio de Salud de Chile, 2010a). Mortality due to diabetes increased between1999 and 2007 from 16.8 to 19.7 per 100,000 inhabitants (17 per cent) (Ministerio de Salud de Chile, 2010a).

Since 2005, the Chilean Ministry of Health has made diabetes management a national priority through federal law within the country's 'Plan for Universal Access with Explicit Guarantees' (i.e. the 'AUGE' Plan). This gives the right to any citizen to receive free healthcare access for early detection, treatment, and self-management support (Ministerio de Salud de Chile, 2010b).

A significant concern arose in the primary care clinics nationwide: *how can primary care centers implement these guarantees for patients with diabetes if the physical infrastructure of most centers is already collapsed and their personnel are overloaded?*

We recognized that there was a significant opportunity for our team at the School of Nursing at Pontificia Universidad Católica de Chile to develop, in collaboration with public primary care centers and the Ministry of Health, tele-care support projects. We also conducted feasibility studies to obtain the evidence which decision makers need to incorporate tele-care as a permanent component of chronic disease management in primary care as a tool to improve chronic disease management without overloading the primary care system.

The purpose of this chapter is to reflect on lessons learned through a sequence of four tele-self-management support projects that the School of Nursing at Pontificia Universidad Católica de Chile (SON) has implemented, between 2004 and 2010, in the commune of Puente Alto, the biggest and one of the poorest communes in Chile. All these projects have had as counterparts the Health Division of the Municipal Corporation of the Commune of Puente Alto, Santiago, and the sponsorship of the Ministry of Health.

I will describe each of these projects because the lessons learned from each one provided information and experience to inform the one that followed. For instance, in our first project we initially did not consider calling cellphones to provide tele-self-management support to patients with type 2 diabetes, as the cost of communication to a cellphone was three times higher than calling a fixed phone. This decision changed very rapidly as we had many inconveniences due to the continuous interruption of the telephone traffic because the copper land lines were stolen, which obliged us to contact our patients through their cellphones. Then we realized that cellphone contacts, although more expensive, were more convenient because we could contact our patients at the first instance at home, at work or in other places outside their home. And that in the long run, the process demanded less professional time, which is scarce and of high cost.

Our effort during these five years has been to develop chronic care strategies for patients with type 2 diabetes, which could be adopted for the care of patients with hypertension and other chronic cardiovascular conditions without overloading the primary care system. In partnership with the health authorities of Puente Alto, we decided to design and try out with patients with type 2 diabetes a tele-self-management support model to improve metabolic control and increase patient satisfaction with the care they receive in primary care centers. The reason we selected diabetes as the prototype chronic disease is that this chronic condition has doubled in Chile in the last ten years. It is also a disease that if not well controlled produces serious health complications, which are of high social and economic impact.

Statistics showed that the prevalence of diabetes in Chile was increasing rapidly from 4.2 per cent in 2005 to 9.2 per cent in 2010. Patients which accessed primary care clinics with high blood glucose levels were not diagnosed in a timely manner nor were they receiving the care they required once it was confirmed that they had diabetes. This is a serious matter because it is known that the early diagnosis of the disease and adequate management reduces the risk of serious complications.

Tele-Self-Management Support: A strategy to improve metabolic control

Several international studies have demonstrated that tele-self-management support, also called tele-care, can contribute to improved metabolic compensation in patients with type 2 diabetes if this strategy is well articulated with face-to-face professional encounters and if telephone protocols and clinical guidelines are used by nurses who are well trained in behavioral change theories (Prochaska and DiClimente, 1984), self-management support strategies and motivational interviewing techniques (Stacey, Noorani, Fisher, Robinson, Joyce, and Pong, 2003; Taylor, Miller, Reilly, Greenwald, Cunning, Deeter, and Abascal, 2003). The tele-self-management support models I describe were selected because they could improve the metabolic control of patients with type 2 diabetes; their satisfaction with care; ability to serve as a natural extension of the traditional primary care model and a desire to identify innovative strategies to use the available human resources without overloading the limited space within the primary care clinics.

We structured and organized the use of tele-self-management support taking into account the characteristics and internal organization of the participating primary care clinics to assure that tele-care would be a natural extension and a supplement to usual care services, which are adequate to treat patients with acute health problems but inadequate to provide care for patients with chronic conditions, such as type 2 diabetes.

The process of refining a tele-care model that would work was accompanied by much frustration for the tele-care nurses of the School of Nursing due to incomplete information in electronic clinical records which was needed to provide personalized and timely self-management support.

It was time to innovate rather than doing more of the same. We agreed with the health authorities of the commune of Puente Alto that we would make every effort to ensure that the pilot initiatives, if successful, would be transformed into institutional programs. This was done to avoid the frequent situation that health centers and patients participate in a chain of isolated pilot projects, which once finished, disappear, because no business plan has been developed as part of the process.

The primary care centers of the commune of Puente Alto have been clinical sites for the students of our School of Nursing for many years. This academic/clinical linkage has been essential. Due to previous community-based projects, our team knew how important it is that the ideas for a project come from the commune rather than from the university. The role of the university is to help to transform these ideas or solutions into a project or research proposal and find the funding for implementation and evaluation. By contrast, with the incorporation of type 2 diabetes in the AUGE plan, the primary care centers would start to be more overloaded than they already were, because patients had now several legal guarantees which include the right to receive timely diagnosis and continuity of care.

However, it was frequent that patients with diabetes, instead of having three professional face-to-face encounters per year, which is the national recommendation, were often seen once a year or less. The reasons were many: a deficit of physicians, high rotation of healthcare providers, patients who had appointments did not show up or they came without having updated lab examinations which are essential to adjust medication doses or provide nutritional feedback, and difficulties of access to the primary care clinic for patients who work, as the centers are not open for diabetes follow-up in the evenings or weekends.

We thought of designing a practice linked and nurse managed tele-support model as a strategy to improve chronic care in general, and particularly for diabetes care. However, no information was available regarding the use of fixed phones and/or cellphones among these patients nor if they would be interested in receiving self-management support by phone as a complimentary activity to the traditional healthcare provided by the primary care center.

With support of students from the School of Nursing and the Institute of Sociology of our University, we did a baseline needs assessment with patients with type 2 diabetes enrolled in public primary care clinics in the commune of Puente Alto. This study had financial support from the Canadian Institutes of Health Research and the Quality Improvement for Complex Chronic Conditions Program from the University of Michigan.

Results showed that over 96 per cent of the patients had either a fixed phone or cellphone or both, and of those reporting access to a telephone, only 6 per cent said that their telephone service was occasionally discontinued due to an inability to pay bills. Many of these patients unsuccessfully attempted to use the telephone as a means to communicate with clinic staff and 60 per cent were interested in receiving self-management support between face-to-face encounters. Patients who had fewer clinic visits were the most likely to report a willingness to receive phone calls in order to enhance their care (Piette, Lange, Issel, Campos, Bustamante, Sapag, Poblete, Tugwell, and O'Connor, 2006). This study confirmed that tele-support could be a real option to improve self-management for patients with type 2 diabetes enrolled in public primary care clinics.

Project 1: Development of a tele-support model to improve self-management

Based on the results of the baseline needs assessment, in 2005, we received a grant from the National Science Fund to design and implement a telephone-mediated

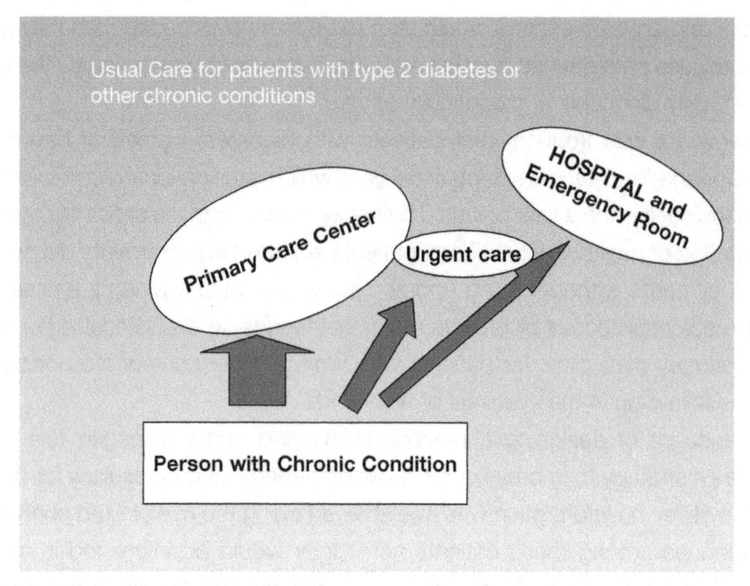

Figure 6.1 Access to healthcare without tele-care

chronic care model – the ATAS model (**A**poyo **T**ecnológico para el **A**utomanejo de Condiciones Crónicas de **S**alud) – to improve self-management, metabolic compensation, and satisfaction with care of patients with type 2 diabetes enrolled in public cardiovascular health programs, as a contribution to the system of universal access with explicit guarantees (AUGE plan). Our counterparts for this project were the Municipal Corporation of Puente Alto, the Ministry of Health, and ENTEL Call Center. A quasi-experimental design was used to evaluate this project.

The ATAS model promotes active participation of patients and family caregivers in health-related decisions and fosters a permanent relationship between the patients and their health services. Nurses who are trained in self-care, behavioral changes, and motivational interviewing use communication technology (for example, phone and the internet) for counseling in chronic disease management in coordination with the patient's primary healthcare team.

The ATAS model has four components: a training program for the primary care clinicians and tele-care team; the tele-counseling service; the self-management tele-support guide; and the software for self-care information, management and follow up (SIGSAC). The first three components are integral parts of the ATAS model. The SIGSAC was developed to be able to implement the ATAS model in the future in other communes of Chile which do not have access to electronic clinical records which are needed to share relevant information between the traditional primary care team and the tele-care nurses.

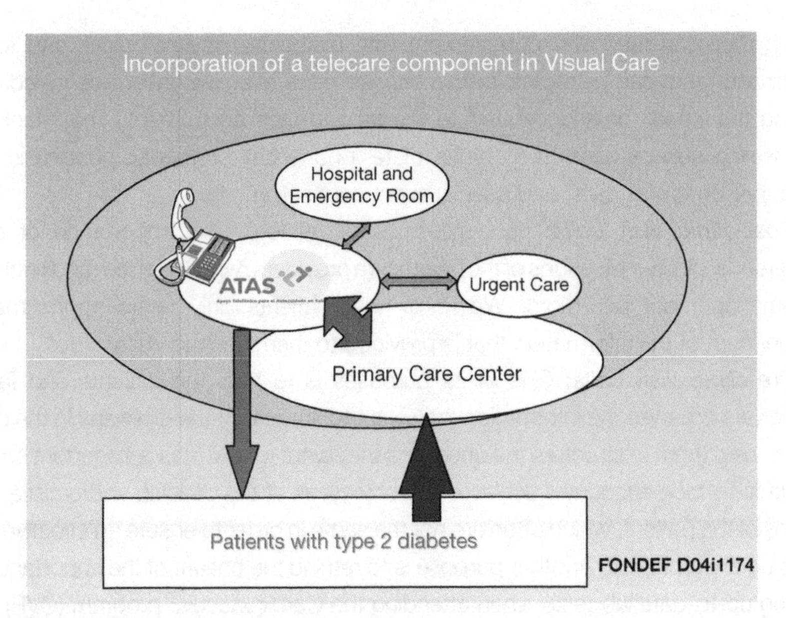

Figure 6.2 A healthcare model with tele-care

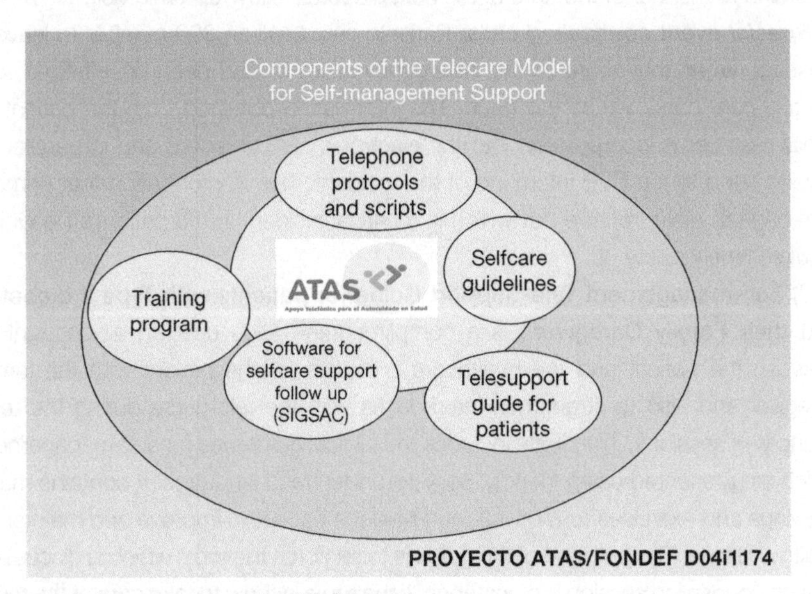

Figure 6.3 Components of the ATAS Model

1) **The Training Program** introduces the primary healthcare team and tele-counseling nurses to the ATAS model and its conceptual framework. This program includes a self-directed learning module.

2) **The tele-counseling** service is the 'heart' of the ATAS intervention. The tele-nurses have access to the electronic health record used by the primary care centers,

which they can read and complement with biological, psychological, and social information that can help clinicians to provide more effective patient-centered care during the limited time dedicated to the face-to-face encounters. The telephone counseling service uses three types of telephone call protocols: post-clinic visit calls, pre-clinic visit calls, and special event counseling calls.

***Post-clinic visit calls*:** Its purpose is to reinforce the importance of drug adherence, clarify indications of the healthcare providers, when needed, and reinforce self-management behaviors. We know that patients only retain approximately 10 per cent of the information that is provided to them in clinic visits.

***Pre-clinic visit calls*:** One of its purposes is to help the patients and family caregivers organize the information they want to share with the clinicians in the clinic and to help them to structure the questions they want to ask. This is important so that the face-to-face encounter achieves the objectives of the clinician and satisfies the needs of the patient, which often are not the same in order to ensure an effective and satisfactory clinic visit. Another purpose is to remind the patient of the importance of having up-to-date lab tests when attending the Cardiovascular program (CVP) and to remind him or her of the date of the next diabetes follow-up clinic visit.

***Special event counseling calls*:** Patients could call an 800 number to leave a message when they went to the emergency room or had been hospitalized and the tele-care nurse would call back. The information obtained from the patient or family member is incorporated into the electronic clinical record and in parallel an email is send to the CVP informing of this incident. This is information that primary care centers never receive but which is a critical incident in the patient's life which requires timely follow up.

3) **Self-management Tele-Support Guide for patients with Type 2 diabetes and their Family Caregivers** is a complimentary guide used in all encounters between the patient and the healthcare providers by the patient with the family caregiver and also to strengthen interactions with the tele-nurse during the tele-counseling sessions. The guide includes the clinical guidelines for self-management which are presented using friendly, easy-to-understand language. It contains many drawings and exercises to motivate and help the patient to improve and maintain a healthy lifestyle. The purpose of the guide is to reinforce the topic which is discussed in each counseling session. For instance, if the topic is 'how to take care of the feet', the nurse would ask the patient to open the guide on the page where foot care is discussed. There is also a space for patients to write comments and questions. This guide is used by tele-care nurses, patients, and family caregivers, as well as by professionals in the primary care center.

4) **Software for self-care information, management and follow up (SIGSAC)** was developed by the Universidad Católica de Chile to facilitate self-management

follow up in healthcare services that do not have access to an electronic medical record.

This project showed that the patients who had access to the ATAS model intervention group; (n = 300 patients) stabilized their blood sugar level, measured by hemoglobin A1c (HbA1c) over a period of 15 months. Whereas the conventionally treated group (n = 306 patients) increased their HbA1c by 1.2 per cent during the same timeframe (Lange, Campos, Urrutia, Bustamante, Alcayaga, Tellez, Pérez, Villarroel, Chamorro, O'Connor, and Piette, J, 2010). The one point difference in the increase of HbA1c, between the intervention and the control group, can predict a 25 percent to 30 percent risk reduction in the intervention group of micro-vascular complications such as retinopathy, neuropathy, renal failure, and amputations in a five to ten year time span (Resnick, 2008).

Also, the intervention group had a significantly higher appointment attendance in the CVP and a reduction in emergency room visits when compared with the control group. Studies show that better appointment attendance predicts better glycemic control in people with diabetes.

Another finding was the significant positive impact of the ATAS model on the self-efficacy in the intervention group versus control group. This is very important because self-efficacy is the best predictor of self-management (Sarkar, Fisher and Schillinger, 2006). There was also a significant increase in client satisfaction with overall care in CVP in the intervention group compared with the control group (Lange, 2007).

Although there were no significant differences identified with regard to reported self-care behaviors between the intervention group and the conventionally treated group, the stabilization of the HbA1c in the intervention group could be explained by two factors: 1) the permanent support of tele-health nurses to assure that patients received the required medication from the health center pharmacy and 2) systematic support to help them adhere to medical treatment.

A common theme identified by tele-care nurses was that patients were more honest and open with them than they were with primary care clinicians regarding their adherence to medication and other self-management behaviors. Patients mentioned that they often did not dare saying the truth to the clinicians (in person) about their difficulties in self-management because they were afraid that the health professionals would get angry.

Dissemination of the findings

To disseminate the findings and increase visibility of the importance of tele-care, we organized a yearly seminar with international experts in chronic disease management, decision support, and tele-care where we also presented the state of advancement of our project. Participants in these seminars includes decision makers from the Ministry of Health, health services, communes, universities, and representatives from the Pan American Health Organization. Faculty members from schools of nursing and medicine, graduate students, clinicians, journalists, representatives from telephone companies and from pharmaceutical laboratories attend these seminars as well. We also facilitated personal interviews between our international experts and the health authorities, which has helped increase interest in our research. The research team also shared its learning and experience through several articles which were published in the main newspapers in Chile. The work and related research has also won the AVONI prize, one of the most prestigious prizes for innovation in Chile, due to its contribution to improve social well-being (Ministerio de Economie 2008).

Project 2: Replication of the ATAS model in Seven primary care centers

Before we had the final results of the ATAS project, the Ministry of Health financed a two-year tele-support implementation project in the seven primary care centers of the commune of Puente Alto. The question the Ministry of Health wanted to answer was if the healthcare providers would be able and willing to make the needed organizational changes to incorporate tele-support as a permanent component of the CVP without increasing resources.

Two thousand patients with type 2 diabetes enrolled in the CVP of these clinics, and benefitted from this model over the course of two years. During this project, we learned that health centers as well as the populations they served had frequent interruptions of their fixed phone services because the copper telephone lines were periodically stolen. Thus, the best way to contact the patients was through mobile phones. The urban population had cellphones with good connectivity that we could use for tele-counseling, even though this is three times more expensive than calling landlines. In the suburban area, the connection of cellphones was of low quality and therefore not appropriate for providing tele-care.

At that point, we had two inconveniences with the use of cellphones for providing tele-counseling: 1) the high cost per minute of traffic and 2) although there was always an appointment set up for tele-counseling, it was not unusual that the patients were not at home at that time but that they answered the phone while shopping, riding in the metro or in other inconvenient places for telephone counseling. After several months, the patients learned that tele-counseling was really helpful for them if they organized themselves to be in a quiet place where they were not interrupted, with their lab results and their tele-support guide. Often family caregivers participated in tele-counseling calls to learn more how to provide self-management support to their significant other with diabetes.

Project 3: Technology transfer of the ATAS model to the commune of Puente Alto

Due to a positive evaluation from the primary healthcare teams as well as from the patients, in 2009 the Ministry of Health funded a one-year project to train a critical mass of health professionals from the healthcare centers in Puente Alto in tele-counseling with emphasis on patient-centered chronic disease management, motivational interviewing, behavior change, self-care, and decision support strategies. Until then, the tele-care service had been provided by trained nurses from our school of nursing who were physically located in the Entel Call Center. Nurses and nutritionists from the seven primary care centers participated in the training program, as presently the urban as well as the suburban areas of Puente Alto have adequate access to cellphones. After the completion of the training program, two of the health centers incorporated tele-counseling as part of their clinical practice. The rest have not, due to time constraints, lack of physical space in the center to provide the tele-counseling sessions, lack of telephone access in the health center, and no lines for cellphone calls. However, several centers are in the process to request equipment and time from their supervisors to be able to provide tele-care at least to the patients who are not well managed.

As the health authorities of Puente Alto are convinced of the benefits of tele-care, we hope that soon the healthcare centers in Puente Alto will be able to act as demonstration sites, where health teams from other communes can learn how to incorporate the ATAS model in the CVP to improve chronic care for patients with type 2 diabetes or other cardiovascular chronic conditions.

Project 4: Mobile phones: Tools to provide support for early diagnosis and self-management for people with type 2 diabetes

Although our tele-care model was well accepted by the healthcare providers as well as by the patients and their family caregivers, one of the criticisms of the decision makers at institutional and ministerial level was that this model could not be easily replicated because it was very expensive due to the need of well-trained nurses who are a very scarce resource in our country. By contrast, the nurses from the School of Nursing who did the tele-counseling during four years realized that a great part of the information and follow-up needs that the patients had could be solved through automated calls and text messages.

This combination of technology could have many benefits. Cellphones do not need copper lines that can be stolen. To receive calls on a cellphone can be done at no cost for the patient. Agreements can be made with telephone companies to reduce the cost of cellphone traffic. Text messages can be sent and read at any point of the day and they have no cost for the person who receives the messages. Messages can be re-read and shared with the family caregivers. This is very important because many patients, especially those who are sixty years and older, have family cellphones and are not used to reading text messages. We tried messages with patients of low socio-economic background and found that although many patients over sixty-five years of age told us that they did not know how to access a text message, they were very interested in learning (especially the women). They also stated that they could receive help from their children or grandchildren who were experts in the use of text messaging.

We also thought that automated calls could be used as reminders as well as to identify if a patient had a special need (for example a patient who is not taking his medicines because of secondary drug effects). In this case, an email could be sent to the particular healthcare center to ask for a personalized follow-up call. With the addition of text messages and automated calls, the professional counseling calls could be reduced significantly. In this way, the human resources and the budget needed for the implementation of such a model would be much lower than the ATAS model that we developed and implemented in Puente Alto between 2005 and 2009 and the chances of dissemination and sustainability higher. This adaptation of the ATAS model is the COSMOS Model (Modelo de **C**omunicación y **S**eguimiento **M**ovil en **S**alud).

The health practitioners from Puente Alto suggested focusing this project on patients with high blood glucose levels to facilitate the process of confirming the diabetes diagnosis in a timely manner. Once a person is diagnosed with type 2 diabetes, she or he will be enrolled in the CVP and will receive self-management support during a three-month period focusing especially on drug adherence, healthy eating, physical activity, and timely clinic visits for diabetes care follow up. The strategies used for self-management support will be telephone counseling, automated calls, text messages, and a tele-support guide for persons recently diagnosed with type 2 diabetes.

The COSMOS project started in August 2010 and was funded for thirteen months by the Mobile Citizen Program of the Inter American Development Bank. We hope that once the whole system is well developed and we have positive evaluations regarding the use of the system as well as its effect on HbA1c, other communes will be able to benefit from this model which will have an open-source software made freely available.

Moving toward national scale

Presently, there are no similar projects in Chile. The only way that a patient can establish contact with the primary care center is by going to the center to get an appointment, and most frequently there will be no appointment available for chronic disease management if she or he has not scheduled two or three months in advance. During the face-to-face encounters very few activities are carried out to activate, empower, and provide self-management support to the patients nor to train the family caregivers. There are several reasons for this, including lack of space, lack of trained health professionals who know how to engage patients with chronic illnesses to increase their perception of self-efficacy, and the fact that healthcare providers are supposed to see a patient with chronic conditions within twenty minutes.

With the technical support of the Pan American Health Organization and the Ministry of Health, our school of nursing recently offered a course, *Evidence Based Chronic Care: a Clinical and Administrative Challenge*. This is an adaptation of the Summer Course Evidence Based Chronic Illness Care offered by PAHO and University of Miami since 2008. Twenty primary healthcare teams (one hundred professionals) working in different areas of Chile were trained. These teams were selected by the Ministry of Health due to their commitment and motivation to improve the care provided to low-income patients with diabetes and hypertension. As a result of this course, each team is designing a project to improve chronic care for their patients, using as their conceptual framework the chronic care model (Wagner, Austin, Davis, Hindsmarsh, Schaefer, and Bonomi, 2001). We hope that the primary care centers where these teams work can act as demonstration sites in the future.

Today, the Ministry of Health is working to define the Sanitary Objectives for the next decade (2011–2020). Due to this experience, there is consensus to incorporate eHealth as a component of the chronic care model for patients with diabetes and hypertension. The question is how to prioritize and use the available resources in order to be as efficient as possible without forgetting that 'no size fits all'. Also, recently, the Ministry of Health has created the concept of a 'Preventive AUGE Plan', which gives us the great possibility to provide the COSMOS model to people with pre-diabetes, as a way to prevent type 2 diabetes.

As Chile has implemented in 2006 an excellent national telephone platform called 'Salud Responde' to provide advice for symptom management and how to navigate through the healthcare system, our team is working with health authorities to provide mHealth self-management support to patients with diabetes who are recently diagnosed. Salud Responde is mostly an inbound call center which mainly provides orientation to people with acute health episodes and help them navigate through the healthcare network. Salud Responde has a triage system with administrative personnel, nurses, and midwives and also physicians twenty-four hours a day, seven days a week. However, to provide chronic care which focuses on behavior changes, special professional skills are needed and healthcare processes have to be standardized. An alliance between Salud Responde and our team at the School of Nursing would be a powerful strategy to provide mHealth self-management support to patients with diabetes, hypertension, and other prevalent chronic conditions.

In synthesis, I envision a national chronic care model that uses the '24/7' platform of Salud Responde to provide self-management support and symptom management recommendations to patients with select chronic diseases through inbound and outbound calls, text messages, and automated calls and that these technologies are well articulated with the care provided by the conventional, face-to-face healthcare network. The decision has to be taken by the Ministery of Health. It is our role to present the advantages of such an alliance.

References

Barceló, A. (2009), 'Evidence Based Chronic Illness Care [Summer Course Booklet]', Miami: University of Miami Miller School of Medicine http://new.paho.org/hq/dmdocuments/2009/ebcic-booklet.pdf [Accessed 15 February 2012].

Lange, I. (2007), Final Report ProyeiFo FONDEF D04i1174 (unpublished).

Lange, I., Campos, S., Urrutia, M., Bustamante, C., Alcayaga, C., Tellez, Á., Pérez, C., Villarroel, L., Chamorro, G., O'Connor, A. and Piette, J. (2010), 'Efecto De Un Modelo De Apoyo Telefónico En El Auto-Manejo Y Control Metabólico De La Diabetes Tipo 2, En Un Centro De Atención Primaria, Santiago, Chile', *Revista Médica de Chile* 138(6): 729–37.

Ministerio de Economia (2008), 'AvoniPremiode Innovation de InteresPublico'

Ministerio de Salud de Chile. (2010a), 'Encuesta Nacional De Salud', http://www.redsalud.gov.cl/portal/url/item/99bbf09a908d3eb8e04001011f014b49.pdf [Accessed July 6, 2012].

Ministerio de Salud de Chile. (2010b), 'Plan Auge', http://www.redsalud.gov.cl/portal/url/page/minsalcl/g_gesauge/presentacion.htm [Accessed July 6, 2012].

Piette, J., Lange, I., Issel, M., Campos, S., Bustamante, C., Sapag, J., Poblete, F., Tugwell, P. and O'Connor, A. (2006), 'Use of Telephone Care in a Cardiovascular Disease Management Programme for Type 2 Diabetes Patients in Santiago, Chile', *Chronic Illness* 2(2): 87–96.

Prochaska, J. and Diclemente, C. (1984), *The Transtheoretical Approach: Crossing Traditional Boundaries of Therapy*, Homewood: Dow Jones Irwin.

Resnick, B. (2008), 'Diabetes Management: The Hidden Challenge of Managing Hyperglycemia in Long-Term Care Settings', *Annals of Long-Term Care* 13(8): 26–32.

Sarkar, U., Fisher, L. and Schillinger, D. (2006), 'Is Self-Efficacy Associated with Diabetes Self-Management across Race/Ethnicity and Health Literacy?', *Diabetes Care* 29(4): 823–9.

Stacey, D., Noorani, H., Fisher, A., Robinson, D., Joyce, J. and Pong, R. (2003), 'Telephone Triage Service: Systematic Review and a Survey of Canadian Call Centre Programs', Ottawa Canadian Coordinating Office for Health Technology Assessment.

Taylor, C.B., Miller, N.H., Reilly, K.R., Greenwald, G., Cunning, D., Deeter, A. and Abascal, L. (2003), 'Evaluation of a Nurse-Care Management System to Improve Outcomes in Patients with Complicated Diabetes', *Diabetes Care* 26(4): 1058–63.

Wagner, E., Austin, B., Davis, C., Hindsmarsh, M., Schaefer, J. and Bonomi, A. (2001), 'Improving Chronic Illness Care: Translating Evidence into Action', *Health Affairs (Millwood)* 20(6): 64–78.

7 Mobile Persuasive Messages for Rural Maternal Health

Divya Ramachandran, University of California, Berkeley

Introduction

Throughout the world and particularly in resource poor settings, women are still dying due to preventable complications in pregnancy and childbirth, a problem almost entirely eradicated in the industrialized world. While conducting research for my dissertation in human computer interaction, I worked on addressing an aspect of this issue by providing a method for delivering clear, persuasive messages about pregnancy and delivery care to mothers-to-be. Specifically, I designed mobile tools to help poorly trained rural health workers establish credibility in their communities as health resources, empowering them to effectively persuade and convince pregnant women and their families to utilize maternal health services even when it conflicts with traditional customs.

Over three years as a graduate student, I conducted field work and iterative design in the poorest state in India, Orissa, which struggles to achieve targeted health outcomes. My particular focus was on Accredited Social Health Activists (ASHAs), who are employed in their own villages by the government to promote free services (like subsidies for institutional deliveries and prenatal care), as well as provide counseling on pregnancy care, family planning, breastfeeding, etc. Through interviews with ASHAs, their trainers, pregnant women and their families, I learned that while ASHAs are employed in most rural villages in India, their training, effectiveness, and acceptance within the village is minimal. ASHAs often spoke of traditional beliefs and rigid social structures that directly opposed the changes that they were tasked to promote.

I experimented with three types of audio-visual aids which could support ASHAs as they communicate with their pregnant clients during house visits and counseling sessions. The first was a series of testimonial videos, recorded by ASHAs themselves on camera phones, which depicted influential village personalities expressing their support of ASHAs. Secondly, I created persuasive videos which were essentially audio-visual versions of textual information found in health handbooks. I observed

ASHAs as they showed these videos to their clients, and found that it took considerable effort to train ASHAs to use the videos effectively by discussing the points in the video, and ensuring that their clients had understood the information. I created a third and final version of the videos which followed a dialogue-based structure, drawing from theories of persuasion, influence, and rhetoric. These videos directly addressed the prevalent myths and barriers which hindered the acceptance and utilization of information and services that ASHAs provided. The videos followed a scripted dialogue, with built-in pauses and questions which ASHAs quickly learned to follow and emulate. I observed a significant increase in the ASHAs' ability to provide effective and high-quality counseling, and considerable engagement from clients and their family members.

My designs were informed by a number of different concepts from theoretical frameworks for persuasion. Throughout the iterative design process, I developed a change model that I pieced together and adapted according to qualitative interviews, lessons from local stakeholders, and iterative field-testing. In this chapter, I describe the evolution of this change model, and the valuable lessons I learned in the process. Six guiding principles for designers of persuasive messages emerged: (1) focus the message on action items, not on broad topics of information, (2) address local myths and barriers, and provide convincing corrections and solutions respectively, (3) create opportunities for structured, persuasive dialogue between humans, keeping in mind that persuasion is a largely social phenomenon in rural communities, (4) include reminders about the positive rewards for changing behavior, paying close attention to local values, (5) capture the most persuasive local language and prosody style, even if it is counterintuitive, and (6) do not assume reactions are honest – persuasion takes time.

Background

Nearly half a million women die each year due to complications in pregnancy and childbirth in developing countries (World Health Organization, 2005). While poor medical facilities, limited transportation means, and scarcity of doctors are still major contributors to these fatalities, it is surprising to observe that barriers imposed by traditional beliefs and customs often prevent women from utilizing free medical services even when they are available. My dissertation research was in the state of Orissa in eastern India, which, as is typical of a number of economically disadvantaged states in India, struggles with improving health outcomes in spite of a number of government and nongovernment efforts.

To improve maternal health in India, the central government has established a National Rural Health Mission, which employs one woman from each village to serve as an Accredited Social Health Activist, or ASHA. ASHAs are charged with promoting free government health services (like subsidies for institutional deliveries, immunizations, and prenatal care), as well as providing counseling on pregnancy care, family planning, breastfeeding, etc. In over two years of qualitative research with ASHAs, pregnant women, their families, and other key community players, I learned that although ASHAs are employed in most rural villages in India, their training, effectiveness, and acceptance within the village is still minimal. Traditional beliefs and rigid social structures limit the change which they promote.

Identifying barriers

I identified a number of barriers to information dissemination and uptake in the communities. Firstly, the structure of the ASHA training programs does not support the acquisition of new knowledge and information. ASHAs attend a monthly sector meeting where they are trained on one new topic each time. In a particular meeting I attended, roughly half of the ASHAs employed in the sector were present. Moreover, the teaching method (formal lectures on a general topic) was not conducive to the ASHAs' education level and schooling experience (they rarely met the eighth grade completion requirement, and many were illiterate). Experienced trainers of health workers from successful NGOs suggested that rather than formal lectures, ASHAs would benefit more from information that is relevant to specific situations that their clients are in as well as instructions on how to effectively share this information with their clients. Secondly, I found that ASHAs had not received training in maintaining an effective work routine. For instance, client monitoring and counseling were aspects unfamiliar to the ASHAs. As a result, the local community did not find the ASHAs as valuable resources and the limited information they could offer was rarely accepted.

Given these challenges faced by ASHAs, I felt that they could be empowered by more effective tools to share health information with their clients. Considering the educational, language, and cultural barriers they needed to overcome, I identified videos on mobile phones as a potentially valuable tool to communicate to clients about what they needed to do in specific health situations. The mobile phone platform was portable, prevalent, and appropriate for ad hoc counseling visits to clients and their families. Videos could convey information comprehensively and consistently in an engaging way for low-literate audiences. Furthermore, as ASHAs shared videos with their clients, they themselves would have the opportunity to learn both factual information and effective counseling techniques over time.

Iterative design of persuasive mobile messages

I created two types of videos: testimonial and persuasive (Ramachandran, Canny, Das, and Cutrell, 2010a). Testimonial videos provided social proof of the ASHA's role and importance. I trained a group of seven ASHAs to record videos using mobile phones and asked them to record messages from influential individuals in their own villages. Their videos featured village leaders, pregnant clients, and even street plays addressing topics including endorsements of the ASHA's role and importance, their own personal health experiences, and instructional messages. These videos provided persuasive social proof to clients that other villagers believed and followed the messages promoted by ASHAs. Persuasive videos were short informative segments about pregnancy-related health issues, which were selected based on prevalence in the target communities. I used relevant content from health handbooks (such as Hesperian Health Guides publications), and adapted these to health advice in line with the local resources and cultural practices with the help of local nurses. A local artist sketched some basic illustrations for the content, and staff at our partner NGO recorded local-language voiceovers. I strung each video together with panning and zooming to give it an animated feel. Each video lasted between thirty seconds and one minute.

I deployed these videos with the seven ASHAs for two months and observed ASHAs using these videos on house visits. Previously, when I had tried to observe ASHAs on house visits, they had been very confused as to what they should actually be doing and kept asking me for instructions. My initial observation when they were now armed with videos was that they provided ASHAs with a concrete example of the information that needed to be disseminated to the client and thus, helped them understand what to accomplish during house visits. However, the videos did not automatically foster conversation, like I had expected. Rather, the ASHA and her clients together watched the videos, and then again asked me for instructions. Therefore, ASHAs had to be trained extensively to use the videos. For instance, I encouraged them to pause the videos, discuss the topics depicted, and engage their clients in conversations about the videos. The effectiveness of the videos depended largely on each individual ASHA's ability to grasp this task of pausing and discussing each topic in the video. I observed that the videos did not seem to ensure any consistency in the quality of counseling.

This experience helped me design a second version of the videos with two important differences. The new version had a built-in dialogue to facilitate client engagement regardless of whether the ASHA was comfortable with this counseling style. The background voiceover asked questions that required yes/no input; the videos automatically paused at these points to facilitate responses and discussion. The second innovation was the use of a persuasive message architecture. I identified prevalent myths and barriers that stopped women from performing particular behaviors and addressed these directly by providing corrections and solutions, respectively.

For example, anemia is a serious problem among rural women, and is the direct cause of one fifth of all maternal deaths (International Institute for Population Sciences and Macro International, 2007). ASHAs distribute free iron tablets to all pregnant women, but many women believe that taking these tablets causes the baby to get too big to deliver normally. A typical lecture-style video modeled off of textual information might present an explanation of iron-deficiency, the risks of anemia and then suggest some actions such as improving diet and taking iron tablets. However, our dialogue-based video opened directly with a question, 'Do you believe that taking iron tablets will cause your baby to get too big, leading to complications during delivery?' This was then followed with a correction, 'That is not true – in fact, iron tablets will give you more strength to get through a normal delivery', and so on. The value of such a dialogic approach was that women immediately related to the topic of the video, and began to discuss this widely believed myth with either the ASHA or others present, and each expressed her opinions on whether it was true. This increased relevance of the message to the client empowered the ASHA to communicate more effectively.

I found that the quality of the counseling session was significantly improved when ASHAs used the new versions of the videos (Ramachandran, Goswami and Canny, 2010b). ASHAs spent more time discussing various aspects of the message, and also elaborated on the message more frequently. From our observations, we found that clients showed more interest and were more attentive when the health worker used the phone messages compared with providing the information orally without the use of videos on the mobile phone.

Identifying the behavior change problem

Early on in my field research, I learned two very important lessons. The first was that I needed to look beyond information access to enable health behavioral changes, and that I should strengthen the persuasive ability of human intermediaries, rather than try to replace them. I elaborate on both these lessons here.

I originally envisioned that the main role of technology would be to enable health information access for rural women. But I found that in all of my interviews with health trainers at NGOs and government health departments, the community health worker model was repeatedly mentioned. Community health workers (like ASHAs) were employed all over the country by various organizations to fill the exact need which I felt technology could address. The question arose as to why the problems were still so prevalent? Rural women had access to all types of information through the health workers, who were, it appeared, trusted, known community members. It was this that prompted my investigation into how ASHAs were actually operating in the field. Upon identifying the many barriers to efficacy they faced, I came to realize that a standalone technology solution did not stand a chance for success in such a complex context. Therefore, I decided to focus my design on **strengthening the existing relationship between the ASHAs and their clients.**

The first thing ASHAs needed, I believed, was access to a pool of correct, relevant health information. At first glance, it appeared that ASHAs already had this. The government was producing pamphlets, handbooks, and flipcharts, and conducting monthly training sessions. As I delved into understanding why the ASHA training program was still producing such inconsistent results, I interviewed a number of freelance or NGO-based health worker trainers, who worked to supplement the broken government training program. It was then that I learned the important lesson that **information access alone is not a solution**, from a seasoned health worker trainer, who explained:

> Just making information available to health workers by no means motivates them to use it. They need to know why to use it, how to use it, why it's personally relevant, and where to utilize it. Only then will it be of any use to them.

This made me realize that I was trying to tackle a twofold behavior change problem. There is a need both to improve the counseling behavior of the ASHAs and to change the health behaviors of their clients. Thus, based on these two important lessons that I learned, I designed the mobile video messages with the belief that a single solution that empowered the ASHAs to become better counselors could improve the health behaviors of their clients.

A mosaic model for behavior change

Upon reflection, it is clear that the change model which I applied for this twofold behavior change problem is a dynamic combination of theoretical principles and empirical evidence. It has evolved greatly, and necessarily so, as throughout this research process, I have had to change and re-evaluate my assumptions. The following is a detailed, chronological, retrospective account of the creation and evolution of my change model.

Mobile solution design

I began with a heavily theoretical approach to persuasion. I studied a number of various theories of persuasion and motivation, such as the theory of planned behavior (Ajzen, 1985), self-efficacy (Bandura, 2006), social influence (Cialdini, 2007), and the Elaboration Likelihood Model (Petty and Cacioppo, 1986). It was unclear which of these (if any) would actually be relevant in the context of rural maternal health. During my in-depth field research, as I interviewed and observed ASHAs, their clients, families, and other stakeholders in the health decision-making process, I looked for signs of relevance of some of these factors. The relevant ones later influenced my design decisions.

For example, it was immediately clear that authorities – in the home, and in the village – had great influence over whether pregnant women utilized the services of ASHAs. That people are more likely to be persuaded by authorities is a factor of social influence, according to the work of Cialdini (Cialdini, 2007). Since authorities varied from village to village, I decided to ask ASHAs to record videos of whomsoever they believed to be authoritative figures in their communities, so that ASHAs could demonstrate the support of these influential persons. Another prevalent factor was the influence of peers, who were also captured in many videos.

I found self-efficacy theory helpful for understanding how to design tools that could motivate ASHAs to become better counselors. Self-efficacy theory revolves around an individual's perception of her own effectiveness with respect to a task (Bandura, 2006). When perceived self-efficacy is high, she will perform tasks well, persisting in the face of obstacles. When it is low, performance is weaker, and she may give up easily in the face of obstacles or acquire avoidance behaviors. Bandura cites the following sources of self-efficacy:

- **Enactive Mastery** is when the subject has a personal experience where she performs a task well, her perceived self-efficacy for that task will improve.
- **Vicarious Experience** is when the subject sees another person have positive outcomes on a task, her perceived self-efficacy will improve.
- **Verbal Persuasion** occurs when an individual hears from another that her performance is good (such as a testimonial), and self-efficacy will improve.

In discussions with ASHAs and their trainers, we identified self-efficacy as a potential problem because the ASHA's environment has many negatives with respect to these three factors. First of all, inadequate training is likely to lead to situations in which ASHAs are unprepared. As quoted earlier, ASHAs also had a hard time assimilating information about situations they had not encountered. Vicarious experience is likely to be poor because ASHAs are quite isolated in their villages. And positive verbal feedback may be rare, while instead the ASHAs receive negative comments since they are regarded as low-status nonexperts by many villagers. I introduced the idea of video testimonials to serve as a form of verbal persuasion, and I designed persuasive videos to provide scaffolding for ASHAs so that counseling would become a concrete task through which ASHAs could demonstrate their expertise in maternal health.

Persuasive message design

Although these theories played a part in guiding my big-picture design ideas, it was not until I started evaluating the videos in the field that I started to understand minor nuances that play an important role in conveying a message persuasively. The design slowly evolved from a one-way standard video, to a structured, dialogic message. In this section, I describe the theoretical underpinnings that guided this evolution, as well as the field experiences.

The science of persuasion through dialogue dates back to Aristotle's classical rhetoric (Lawson-Tancred, 1991). Particularly relevant are his writings on *logos*, or the persuasive power of a speech based on its ability to prove a truth, or apparent truth, through practical arguments. Rather than rely on logic, logos-based arguments appeal to the listener's practical reasoning, presenting the desired action as a direct implication of the listener's own salient beliefs. I also reviewed some common practices in the field of public health and their underlying models for designing health messages (Maibach and Parrot, 1995).

Health messages should:

1. Appeal to the listener's self-efficacy, or perceived ability to perform an action by recommending simple and achievable actions (Bandura, 2006);
2. Induce behavior change by addressing the underlying set of salient beliefs that cause a specific behavior (Ajzen, 1985);
3. Maximize involvement of and personal relevance to the listener to encourage more lasting attitude change, according to the elaboration likelihood model of persuasion, this happens through central processing of the message (Petty and Cacioppo, 1986), and
4. Use positive effective appeals to arouse more positive feelings and acceptance toward the recommended action (Maibach and Parrot, 1995).

With some initial ideas from these theories, I designed dialogic messages and iterated on them in the field. The following features of the messages proved to be critical. Under each feature, I have referenced the relevant theory above. For simplicity, I use the example iron-deficiency anemia as the main issue to be addressed.

Actions as Key Takeaways: The first video messages I designed were based directly on text, and so they were focused on a particular topic or subheading of a chapter (for example anemia). But I observed that when pregnant women and ASHAs watched video messages based directly off of text, they could only recall concrete actions, and not specific details, especially when the messages contained multiple conditional statements. Therefore, the new messages were focused mainly on the desired action (such as take iron pills), with an explicit *action* described in simple steps to improve self-efficacy. The action was repeated multiple times in each message.

Culturally Relevant Arguments: Through discussions with ASHAs and pregnant women, I learned that women do not take their iron tablets for a number of reasons, many of which are based on traditional myths (for example, the baby will get too big to deliver normally), or social barriers (for example mother-in-law does not allow her to take extra vitamins). I categorized the arguments used by women against these actions into the two types: **myths** and **barriers**. Addressing these specific relevant arguments was critical for an effective persuasive message, according the theory of planned behavior.

I constructed the argument using a simple formula. For each action, there are a number of associated myths and barriers. They are first presented in this way:

- **[Myth-Correction-Action]** A widely believed *myth* is introduced and immediately followed by a *correction* to that myth. This is followed by a recommended *action*.
- **[Barrier-Solution-Action]** A relevant *barrier* is addressed, followed by a *solution* for dealing with that barrier, followed by a recommended *action*.

Dialogic Structure: Keeping the basic content constant, I designed the messages in two styles, building on my previous research (Ramachandran and Canny, 2008) and the elaboration likelihood model (Petty and Cacioppo, 1986). I hypothesized that audio-visual messages that require direct response from the user are more persuasive than longer lecture-style recitations of information (as is often used when moving from text to audio-based presentation). In order to enforce user responses in the dialogic version, we inserted *rhetorical question tags* after each piece of information, which elicited a 'yes' or 'no' response from the user. Our message architecture differentiates between lecture and dialogic style messages. The figure below shows how myths and barriers are presented in both styles.

In a study which compared the use of the lecture style and the dialogic, I found that the dialogic messages provided more scaffolding for the health workers, resulting in more consistent, high-quality counseling behavior (Ramachandran *et al.*, 2010b). Specifically, I measured a statistically significant difference ($p < 0.001$)

	Lecture	Example	**Dialogic**	Example
Myth	General Statement	*Many women believe that <myth>.*	Question about personal beliefs	*Do you believe that <myth>?*
Correction	Explanation	*<myth> is not true; in fact, <correction>.*	Explanation with rhetorical question tags	*<myth> is not true; in fact, <correction>, did you know that?*
Action	Instruction	*You should <action>.*	Request for personal commitment	*Will you <action>?*
Barrier	General Statement	*Many women face <barrier>.*	Question about personal beliefs experience	*Do you ever face <barrier>?*
Solution	Suggestion	*If you ever face <barrier>, you can <solution>.*	Instruction with rhetorical question tags	*If you ever face <barrier>, you can <solution>, okay?*
Action	General Instruction	*You should <action>.*	Request for personal commitment	*Will you <action>?*

Figure 7.1 Lecture and dialogic approaches
Note: Table reprinted from Ramachandran *et al.*, 2010b; copright held by Authors.

in the quality of counseling, measured by the time spent in discussions of the message between the ASHA, her client and bystanders, as well as the frequency of explanations by the ASHAs during breaks and pauses. However, as is discussed later, I have not yet successfully measured the impact of this improved quality on health behaviors.

Positive Rewards: After presenting corrections and solutions to all the relevant myths and barriers, I included a short message that reminded the listener of the positive rewards of performing the action. In this case, taking iron pills would make the baby stronger, and the mother would have a happy, healthy child. I found during my interviews that focusing on the health of the baby, rather than the health of the mother was more effective, especially with other influential family members like the mother-in-law of the pregnant woman.

Local Language and Prosody: I selected a tribal site for evaluating these messages, and felt initially that messages should be in the local tribal language, Kui, rather than the common local language, Oriya. However, I found that many of the ASHAs were not tribal, and therefore could not speak or understand Kui and only spoke Oriya. Therefore, I recorded the messages in both languages (by the same speaker), and implemented a language toggle button so that both ASHAs and their tribal clients could understand the message.

There was no way I could record the messages by a professional voice actress, as it would be impossible to find one who could speak Kui. I found a young school teacher who spoke both Kui and Oriya, but I felt her style sounded too rehearsed, and lacked emotion. I kept trying to push a more natural prosody, as I felt that would be more persuasive. My local contacts insisted on the simpler style. I came to realize that what they were suggesting was simply more culturally appropriate, and observed the immense impact of the messages when I piloted them. As one NGO staff remarked, 'Tribals are simple people: they don't need emotion, they just need a clear message'. This was a very important and unexpected lesson.

Response Behavior: I had imagined that the dialogic message structure would enable a very effective feature – to branch to relevant messages based on the response of the pregnant woman (for example, if a woman said she did not believe a particular myth, the correction would be skipped, and next myth or barrier would be introduced). However, during my initial pilots, I realized that responses were not always honest; they did not always admit to believing a myth or facing a barrier. For example, one participant insisted after every message element that none of them applied to her and that she took iron pills daily. However, when the ASHA asked her to show her the pills, the participant could not find them. One interpretation is that she was trying to present herself as socially acceptable, as reported by other researchers who studied survey responses that were directed to a health worker with a mobile device (Cheng, Ernesto and Truong, 2008). Therefore, I decided that regardless of the response, no messages should be skipped.

Measuring persuasion

All too often in the mHealth space, it seems that technology solutions are designed with little or no evaluation of their impact on health. Specifically in the area of health information, few evaluations exist still seem to measure increased knowledge, rather than behavior change. This is not surprising, since knowledge is much easier to measure. But this is not a metric for behavior change, but one for information access, and these two must be distinguished from each other.

As mentioned earlier, in my evaluation of dialogic mobile messages, I was unable to statistically prove that women changed their behaviors due to the improved efficacy of ASHAs. There are a number of reasons why I believe that I could not, and these are detailed in another publication (Ramachandran *et al.*, 2010b). First of all, I was limited by the logistics of accessing and recruiting a sufficient number of ASHAs because they are vastly spread out in rural areas. This resulted in a great variability among the ASHAs, where some were extremely sincere, and others less motivated. Second, even with these few ASHAs, it appeared that the community (caste) from which they hailed might have influenced their persuasive power. This demonstrates the sensitivity of the measure of persuasion to various factors in the environment, be they social, cultural, or political. Finally, I was limited in the amount of time I could spend in the field, but persuasion takes time. I strongly believe that some effect could be measured if I had the resources (time, manpower, and money) to run a longer-term study with more participants. Surprisingly, even with so much interest and investment in mHealth, very little of it is being spent on evaluation. I believe we have reached a stage where we really need to be producing proof that these investments are in fact affecting health behaviors and outcomes.

Guidelines for creating persuasive messages

Despite having studied a number of different theoretical frameworks, I found that no single one perfectly fit in the context in which I was working. What worked best for me was a sort of mosaic model, which pieced together different proven principles, with some tweaks to adapt the concepts appropriately to the context, and which I adapted and developed over time in response to what I observed in the field. My change model has evolved with my designs, but has been an integral part of them; I believe some mix of theory, practice, and intuition is necessary for creating an appropriate behavior change model in any context, as there are a number of factors that can influence the persuasive power of any interaction, be it human-to-human, or human-to-machine.

As a summary for anyone skimming through this chapter, the following are the important lessons that I learned, that I feel would be valuable for anyone designing persuasive messages for promoting healthy behaviors:

- Focus the message on action items, not on broad topics of information.
- Address local myths and barriers, and provide convincing corrections and solutions, respectively.
- Create opportunities for structured, persuasive dialogue between humans, keeping in mind that persuasion is still a largely social phenomenon in rural communities.

- Include reminders about the positive rewards for changing behavior, paying close attention to local values.
- Capture the most persuasive local language and prosody style, even if it is counterintuitive.
- Do not assume reactions are honest; persuasion takes time.

References

Ajzen, I. (1985), 'From Intentions to Actions: A Theory of Planned Behaviour', in J. Kuhl and J. Beckmann (eds), *Action Control: From Cognition to Behaviour*, Heidelberg: Springer: 11–39.
Bandura, A. (2006), 'Guide for Constructing Self-Efficacy Scales', in F. Pajares and T. Urdan (eds), *Self-Efficacy Beliefs of Adolescents*, Greenwich: Information Age Publishing 5: 307–37.
Cheng, K., Ernesto, F. and Truong, K. (2008), *Participant and Interviewer Attitudes toward Handheld Computers in the Context of HIV/AIDS Programs in Sub-Saharan Africa*. ACM CHI 2008 Conference on Human Factors in Computing Systems, Florence, Italy, ACM.
Cialdini, R. (2007), *Influence: The Psychology of Persuasion*, New York: Harper Collins.
International Institute for Population Sciences and Macro International (2007), '2005–2006 National Family Health Survey, India (Nfhs-3)', http://www.nfhsindia.org/nfhs3.html [Accessed 15 February 2012].
Lawson-Tancred, H. (1991), *The Art of Rhetoric*, New York: Penguin Group.
Maibach, E. and Parrot, R. (1995), *Designing Health Messages: Approaches from Communication Theory and Public Health Practice*, Thousand Oaks, CA: Sage Publications.
Petty, R. and Cacioppo, J. (1986), *Communication and Persuasion: Central and Peripheral Routes to Attitude Change*, New York: Springer.
Ramachandran, D. and Canny, J. (2008), 'The Persuasive Power of Human-Machine Dialogue', in H. Oinas-Kukkonen (ed) *Persuasive '08 Proceedings of the 3rd International Conference on Persuasive Technology*, Heidelberg: Springer-Verlag: 189–200.
Ramachandran, D., Canny, J., Das, P. and Cutrell, E. (2010a), *Mobile-Izing Health Workers in Rural India*. CHI 2010, ACM Press.
Ramachandran, D., Goswami, V. and Canny, J. (2010b), *Research and Reality: Using Mobile Messages to Promote Maternal Health in Rural India*. International Conference on Information and Communication Technologies and Development.
World Health Organization (2005), *World Health Report: Make Every Mother and Child Count*, Geneva: World Health Organization.

8 MOTECH

Jessica Osborn, Grameen Foundation—Ghana

MOTECH project description

The Mobile Technology for Community Health (MOTECH[1]) Initiative is a partnership between the Ghana Health Service, Grameen Foundation, and Columbia University's Mailman School of Public Health, with funding from the Bill & Melinda Gates Foundation. The project uses two interrelated mobile phone applications to increase the quantity and quality of antenatal and neonatal care in rural Ghana with a specific goal of improving health outcomes for mothers and their newborns.

Access to basic health information in rural areas of Ghana is extremely limited, resulting in lack of knowledge about maternal and child health, low uptake of health services, and adherence to often-damaging local myths and cultural practices. This contributes to high maternal and child morbidity and mortality. Therefore, MOTECH has developed the '**Mobile Midwife**' application which enables pregnant women and their families to receive SMS or prerecorded voice messages on personal mobile phones that provide time-specific information about their pregnancy each week. Information is provided in the client's local language and is localized to address issues faced in various regions of the country. The messages continue through the first year of life of the newborn and reinforce well-child care practices and vaccination schedules.

There is also a '**Nurse Application**' that enables Community Health Nurses to electronically record care given to patients and identify women and newborns in their area who are due for care. Previously, this data was collected and aggregated on paper owing to shortage of power and computers in rural health facilities. This resulted in inaccurate data and time delays, so reducing its value for decision makers.

Using the former paper-based system, it was also difficult for nurses to identify clients overdue for care since data was collected in up to thirty different registers. Therefore, MOTECH has linked its two mobile applications so that if a patient has missed treatment that is part of the defined care schedule, the Mobile Midwife service sends an **appointment reminder** to the patient and nurse.

The MOTECH system was launched in July 2010 in one district in the Upper East Region of Ghana and has registered over 7,000 pregnant women and children under five. To validate the replicability of the service, expansion to a district in

Central Region was scheduled for June 2011. A randomized controlled trial in the Upper East Region would be completed by Columbia University in November 2011 to determine the impact of the intervention on health outcomes. In this chapter, we will explore some of the lessons learned in the process of developing these mobile applications, examining each individually.

Prior lessons learned

Grameen's earlier work on Google SMS and early testing of an IVR application in Uganda had equipped us with a lot of understanding about how to develop technology solutions for the poor. This knowledge included skills in effective product development processes and methodologies. For instance, we honed our skills in 'rapid prototyping' – quickly testing very early instances of a product with hundreds of users, incorporating learnings gained from this exercise into the service efficiently, and continuing to develop the product with users directly in an iterative process of testing and application modification. The Uganda experience also provided us with a good comprehension of user needs and preferences in sub-Saharan Africa; we had already made mistakes which had questioned and tested certain assumptions, so we did not need to make those same mistakes again. For example:

- We knew that SMS is not the optimal channel for reaching the poor (we had found that even among those who were literate in English or local languages, the depth of comprehension of a message was far more superficial when information was delivered in text compared with voice).
- We knew that rural clients in particular struggle to navigate an IVR system even when directions are provided in local languages.
- We knew that mobile use is of a fluidity which precludes using phone number as an identifier (users have multiple SIMs and different phones are used when batteries are down which is a frequent occurrence when power sources are scarce).
- We had tried and failed to charge rural poor users a nominal fee for information services.
- We had learned that in many African cultures, people go by several different names which are sufficiently interchangeable and have enough accepted alternative spellings that we would need to enable broad search algorithms when trying to locate clients in a database.

Some validation testing was needed to confirm that these factors were applicable in Ghana as they were in Uganda (for the most part they were), but overall our prior experience enabled us to start our product designs at a later stage of maturity.

A key lesson learned in this process of transferring skills and knowledge between countries and projects was simply realizing the importance of capitalizing on these prior experiences. Beyond circulating the human capital that has gained this experience, how can an organization ensure to document and systematize learnings in such a way that they are retained and are useful to subsequent innovations while still enabling the agility and perspicacity in *new* challenges that is needed for success? This is an element on which we as an organization continue to work, through honest and frank documentation of challenges as well as successes, and through open communication of these across our own projects and externally – being as open source with our ideas and experiences as we intend to be with our code.

Despite the 'head start' that our prior experiences lent us, MOTECH is focused on a narrower domain than our previous work; it introduced us to a new end-user, the healthcare worker, and it took us deeper down the paths of using voice and mobile forms as channels for disseminating and collecting information, respectively. Therein lay plenty of new discoveries for us, some of which we will share here.

'Mobile Midwife': Application for pregnant women and their families

Assumptions

The number of mobile phone subscriptions is increasing rapidly worldwide (ITU, 2009), particularly among low- and middle-income groups, including those in Ghana (AudienceScapes, 2009). Grameen's work in mobile applications begins with a desire to use this ever-expanding network of mobile phones as a platform for dissemination of information to those who currently have least access to it, the poor, with the intention that this information might enable them to improve their livelihoods.

As limited as information access may be particularly in rural areas, there have been various important and valuable efforts in social and behavior change communication (BCC) in these areas: informative posters, community radio, theater, infomercials, peer education, advocacy, and use of key community informants are just some of the methods that have been useful in conveying health information at the community level. We started the project with the belief that the communication of this information through mobile would introduce depths of both personalization and share-ability that cannot be achieved through these other mediums.

- *Share-ability:* In testing we found that users liked being able to access their messages at any time and being able to play them as many times as they liked, allowing them to share messages with friends and relatives.
- *Personalization:* Health information which is tailored to the individual receiving it – their stage in pregnancy, care history, location, local value system, and preferences for *when* and *where* they access advice – is a level of information tailoring and ease of access that has not been available in these communities to date. When we look to the likes of Amazon, Google advertising, and Facebook, it seems that their successes partially lie in how intrinsically well they know their clients and how information is tailored so specifically to them. Applying this to the health domain requires confidentiality and sensitivity of a different league, but we believe that the principle remains the same – offering information which is personally relevant to the client is likely to make them listen up. Doing this requires building technology which can support it: a message engine which determines how many weeks pregnant someone is, what care they are (over)due for, what region they are from, which language they speak, and aligning this and other metadata in order to select the appropriate message to be sent. This is challenging, but just the beginning. Having determined what we believed to be the appropriate technology, we then needed to test our assumptions with real users.

Early research and product testing

We conducted a Mobile Health ethnography to assess the state of information, communication, and mobile phone use for maternal and newborn health within both the health sector and the general population (Mechael, 2009). This showed us that there was significant demand for maternal health information among the general population and readiness from these groups to receive such information through the mobile phone. The report also highlighted practices which lead to maternal and neonatal morbidity and mortality, some of which could potentially be ameliorated through information delivered through a mobile phone. For instance, the ethnography identified delay in receiving care and low uptake of services as a contributor to poor health, which could be countered through education in problem recognition, explanation of the benefits of seeking health services, and reminders to attend the health facility for certain care appointments. The ethnography also highlighted the extent to which local myths and traditions can negatively affect the health of an expectant mother and also dictate care seeking practices during pregnancy. This report, therefore, gave us some ideas about the types of content that would be useful and also the kinds of challenges we should expect. We were particularly nervous about the effect that strong local traditions could have on the uptake of any mobile services we might develop, and the extent to which people might trust information delivered through such a medium; could information delivered through an intensely modern medium be trusted enough to call into question myths and traditions that have existed for centuries?

With this background, we then sketched out a product idea: a service which sends information to women each week of their pregnancy, including appointment reminders tailored to their personal care history. We wanted to quickly test out if this would be of interest to our target audience, if they would find information delivered through the mobile phone trustworthy and accessible and if users would prefer information through SMS or voice. To do this, we set up a basic hotline, with qualified health professionals manning lines between 9 a.m. and 5 p.m. on the days of field testing. Three field teams went out on each day to broadcast awareness of the service, assess user satisfaction with responses, and profile potential users.

- Two-hundred and thirty-six queries from over 220 participants were received in three days.
- The demand for information and level of interest in the service were far greater than expected and overstretched the capacity of the three operators to answer calls quickly enough. The participants wrote down the hotline number and tried to call through the night, although opening hours were clearly communicated. Some participants were willing to spend their own units on making calls to the hotline. News of the hotline spread so that calls were received from communities outside of the prototyping area. On the whole, we saw huge demand for health information and saw that the participants were delighted to receive this information and seemed comfortable obtaining it through a mobile phone.
- One single query was received through SMS, indicating to us the importance of providing information through voice.
- We were surprised that almost 20 percent of those calling for information were men, who seemed to like the private and confidential aspect of the mobile medium. This made us realize a potential to target information to men as well as pregnant women.
- Although we advertised the service as a pregnancy hotline, 62 per cent of queries were related to child health. This encouraged us to consider extending an information service through the child's first year.

- The exercise taught us some valuable lessons about the operational aspects of delivering content through mobile. Many calls dropped mid-conversation in poor network areas and especially during rain storms, teaching us that we needed to build a service which enabled people to call back into retrieve their messages.
- The sheer volume of questions received taught us a lot about people's knowledge gaps, guiding us in the right direction for content development.

Getting the content right

One of our content partners, BabyCenter, a trusted source of online pregnancy information for millions of people around the world, says one of the keys to really good content is getting it 'remarkably right'; knowing exactly what someone is going through at just the right time and offering clear advice for how to deal with it.

Creating content that we were confident was 'remarkably right', actionable, simple, localized, and medically sound took many rounds of consultations with potential end-users, health practitioners, policymakers, and local and global development partners.

We started by asking some pregnant women and their husbands to keep diaries; we provided them with voice recorders into which they were encouraged to record their thoughts, experiences, challenges, and questions related to pregnancy. Through this, we learned how many people are influential in a single pregnancy: mothers-in-law, grandmothers, husbands, and even landlords are significant in decision making during a woman's pregnancy in the Upper East Region of Ghana, with the opinions of pregnant woman herself often being relegated. Perhaps influenced by Western models of pregnancy being a deeply personal experience for a couple, this aspect was a new learning for us as an organization. We realized that we needed to target a broader range of actors as recipients of 'Mobile Midwife' and the information it delivers. We needed to understand the experiences of the pregnant woman in order to reinforce her voice in the household, and provide actionable advice that was targeted not only to the pregnant woman and her husband, but also to others in the family. We initially thought of having different information channels for different actors, but realized that a single phone is usually shared among the household, so this would not really work. We then realized that the way that phones are shared might therefore be an advantage since the health message might be heard by any actor depending on who had the phone at the time at which it was sent. Since the person who hears the message is likely to be one of the actors with influence on the pregnancy, the information, if sufficiently broad, would also be of relevance to them and could therefore also benefit the pregnancy.

Through the pregnancy diaries, we also found that pregnant women in particular expressed a huge demand for information, but also for advice, encouragement, and reassurance. This made us see the product we were developing in a different light – we were not developing a catalogue of facts but rather a friend or auntie to whom people could turn for trusted advice. We believed that enabling the service to take on this role would make people have more trust in the more factual content provided.

Next we held focus groups with other actors who are influential during pregnancy, exploring their beliefs, knowledge gaps, attitudes toward a pregnancy including their fears, challenges, and joys. These focus groups enabled to develop content which could talk to the information needs of each group. For instance, we learned that where women felt that men prevented them from seeking healthcare because they did not appreciate the medical need for it, most men actually explained that they did not have enough money to enable their wives to go to the facility and were worried about that because they realized the importance of such visits medically. This was reported to be a common source of household tension. Having knowledge of subtle dynamics such as this enabled us to create messages which acknowledged constraints and tried to provide tips on how to overcome them (for instance, explaining that healthcare for pregnant women is free; many men were not aware of this).

From these focus groups, we realized that we would not only need to translate content into different Ghanaian languages, but also need to localize *content* for different cultures within the country, since traditional beliefs, myths, and cultural practices in particular are highly variable between regions. We are now determining scalable ways of localizing through identifying a core curriculum of content which remains the same between regions into which localized content is inserted at predetermined points, and developing light and efficient mechanisms for gathering localization information for each area of the country.

Finally, lengthy consultation with health practitioners, policymakers, and local and global development partners ensured that information provided was in line with Ghana Health Service priorities and care protocols.

Once we developed our content, the process of translating and recording it brought out some interesting lessons. We knew from Uganda and our own experiences as users that for voice applications the sound of the voice is important. Therefore, we tested different voices with many potential users. Surprisingly, we found that women were quite open to receiving information from a male voice for certain topics such as those about savings and finances, support that pregnant women might need during pregnancy, and some childcare messages. Indeed, many said they were happy about that since their husbands might be encouraged to become equally knowledgeable and supportive as the man reading the message. We also found that, consistent with people seeing the service as a source of reassurance and advice, people wanted to hear an older, soft voice, like a trusted, experienced and sympathetic 'auntie' (a term used in Ghana to show respect toward elders). Once we had found actors who spoke the appropriate languages, there was concern from users about the 'depth' of their accent. Consistent with research on source credibility, users disliked voices with accents from 'deep in the village' as they were not trusted as being knowledgeable enough (Erickson, Lind, Johnson, and O'Barr, 1978; Sternthal, Dholakia and Leavitt, 1978; Heesacker, Petty and Cacioppo, 1983; Pornpitakpan, 2004). Equally voices who sounded too educated were not accepted, as they were not seen as being from a place that would enable them to fully understand the daily struggles of life in the users' area.

Messages were diligently translated and back translated, and we even spent time finding symbols in the word processor which were needed to express the local languages in written form. However, when it came to recording these we were not able to find anyone – across all levels of education – who could read the translations, except for professional translators, and local language linguistics experts. With hindsight it makes perfect sense: these are oral languages whose written forms have not been extensively developed. After weeks dedicated to obtaining the perfect written translations, we had to abandon the written local language scripts and resort to impromptu translations from the English text by the voice actors themselves, in consultation with a qualified health worker fluent in the language.

Mobile access

Mobile phone ownership in Ghana is estimated to be around 32 per cent, with 72 per cent of people estimated to have access through someone in their household (AudienceScapes, 2009). Even for those who own a phone, SIMs are frequently changed if a stronger signal can be received with one network over the other, so there is often not one single phone number on which someone can be reached. Therefore, we designed the system to enable calls and SMSs to be pushed out to those who had reliable access to a phone, but which also enabled all subscribers to call in to access their messages. Relying on women calling in to retrieve their messages, however, has resulted in lower uptake of the messages overall. Since IVR systems are not often used in Ghana, some women find navigating them challenging, even with directions provided in local languages, so this may be a barrier to uptake of this option. Even if a household owns a phone, it may be switched off frequently as charging phones is challenging in rural areas. Therefore, we designed the system to keep attempting to call a phone until it is turned on. Interestingly, when registering clients, we found that many who had a phone in their household did not know the phone number from memory. Therefore, when organizing registration days and in marketing collateral we asked people to make sure to bring their phone number (if they had one) with them written down for registration.

Personal identifiers

The issue of how to uniquely identify clients was challenging to resolve. There is no comprehensively executed national ID system currently in place in Ghana and no universally implemented identifiers used in the health system. However, for Mobile Midwife we needed an identifier or combination of identifiers that could be easily remembered or located by the patient, and easily entered onto a phone keypad and processed by an IVR-type system to identify the patient uniquely when they call in to retrieve messages. We considered using phone number as a way to identify clients calling in to MOTECH, but realized that this would not work owing to the high turnover of different SIM cards and the widespread practice of sharing phones meaning that more than one MOTECH client may be relying on a single SIM.

After some investigation, we realized that developing an ID scheme for MOTECH would be necessary for accurate data and ease of access. Therefore, all clients registered in the system are issued a nine-digit numeric code at registration, which takes place at a health facility or by calling a toll free call center. We selected a numeric code to enable easy input using a phone keypad. The client is provided with this number on an ID card which is issued at registration, or over the phone for call center registrations. This ID number is also noted by health workers next to the client's record in their registers. The ID number is used from then on by both the nurse and the client. When nurses enter information about a particular patient into the MOTECH system, they use the patient's ID number. When a patient calls in to MOTECH to retrieve their messages, they are first requested to select their language, and then they are asked, in their selected language, to enter their MOTECH ID number. Entering the ID number tells the system who the client is, enabling their personalized message to be played.

Another challenge was designing a methodology for identifying duplicate registrations in the MOTECH database, or uniquely identifying patients in the case that their MOTECH ID has been lost. Using simple demographic fields such as name and date of birth seemed unreliable since our clients often go by several different names and are not so concerned with accurate spelling of them. Also, many people in rural areas do not know their date of birth. The only solution to this issue has been to rely on a triangulation of fields to try to identify patients: a broad search is enabled when trying to locate a patient in the database by name, and a combination of address, date of birth (where possible), National Insurance Number (where possible), and relation to other family members (for example children) in the database are all relied upon for unique identification. This system has worked quite well, although it has not been able to eliminate the instances of duplicate records altogether; manual review is still required to identify some cases.

Accidental learning

The intended design for the system was that a user who wants to retrieve their messages by calling MOTECH would call a toll free, universal short code which would connect them with our IVR system. We were not able to set up this toll free, universal code in time for launch so as an interim solution we had to connect through a normal phone number which charges at peer-to-peer rates. In order to be able to offer this service free of charge to our users under this set up, we designed the system to respond to a 'flash'[2] from a client (Donner, 2009). 'Flashing' prompts the system to call the user back, placing them in the IVR home menu. Although we intended this to be a temporary solution, from initial focus groups with users it seems that they really like being able to flash the system. Flashing is a widely used mode of communication in Ghana, so people are familiar with it. Most of all, users like that with flashing they can be sure that they will not be charged for the call.

MOTECH nurse application

Nurses in rural clinics in Ghana currently rely on a substantial number of patient registers for data collection, sometimes up to thirty different registers can be used in one facility. Some are provided by the Ghana Health Service, others are simple exercise books formatted by nurses themselves. Different registers are used for different care types (for example outpatients, antenatal care, postnatal care, delivery, and child welfare). There are challenges with this mode of data collection.

Firstly, it is difficult to link different types of care for an individual patient to see their care history. For example, you cannot see from the antenatal register which sicknesses a woman has suffered from during her pregnancy.

Secondly, nurses have to spend a lot of time (four to six days per month) aggregating data in the registers to complete reports that they are required to send monthly to the district offices, and which are subsequently aggregated for the district and region. Not only is this process extremely time consuming for nurses, but its manual nature also makes it very error prone, reducing the usefulness of the data for decision-making, monitoring, and reviewing performance.

Thirdly, although the nurse spends a lot of time extracting information from the registers to send to managers further up the system, very little useful information flows back to the nurse. For instance, it is extremely difficult, using the registers, to identify clients who have defaulted for care or who are high risk for certain illnesses.

It seems clear that transaction-level electronic recordkeeping would combat many of these challenges. Some projects and research have attempted to address this challenge by providing facilities with laptops (Fontelo, Liu, Zhang, Ackerman, and Tolentino, 2008) (Partners in Health, EngernderHealth, Better Health Outcomes through Mentoring and Assessment), or smartphones (Open Data Kit, eMOCHA, Sene Project) for data dissemination, capture, and submission for healthcare providers. While such initiatives undoubtedly add value, we wanted to try a solution using lower-end technology which would be more manageable for government entities to support in terms of training, power, and hardware costs.

Selecting handsets and mode of data transmission

We set out with a goal to rely on nurses' existing phones. A poll of over 100 nurses' phones in the Upper East Region showed that only around 15 per cent of them had Java-enabled phones, making reliance on nurses' phones synonymous with reliance on an SMS or voice solution for data transmission. Therefore, we trialed an SMS-based system, which revealed a number of challenges:

- Older nurses in particular did not know how to send or retrieve SMS, so induction had to include basic SMS lessons in addition to data entry training.
- Even those nurses proficient with SMS struggled to follow the strict syntax required to compile a structured SMS – typos, missing spaces, and incorrect data order made data capture difficult. We tried to overcome this by saving SMS templates containing field titles on to the phone as SMS drafts. This did not work in many instances, since the low memory capacity of many of the phones put a limit on the number of SMSs that could be saved as drafts, and yet there were around ten different SMS types that were required for our purposes.
- Some phones did not have a drafts folder. In these cases, we saved the messages in the inbox, but again here we were met with the challenge of low SMS storage capacity.
- We also found that nurses accidentally edited the SMS templates, meaning that subsequent submissions were flawed.
- Some phones were not able to send SMS because Message Center settings were incorrect.

Providing training to overcome these challenges was extremely challenging when supporting the many different handset types owned by nurses.

In addition to these data challenges, there were several social aspects which made using nurses' own phones impossible. Phone access and ownership seemed to be as fluid among nurses as it was among people in the community. Many nurses shared phones with family members, so there would be times when no phone was available in the clinic, and the fact that phones were lent to non-Ghana Health Service staff posed a privacy risk for patient data. Lack of charging solutions was also an issue, as not all facilities had reliable power. Finding a charging solution for the many different phone types that nurses were using would have proven challenging. Furthermore, nurses were unsatisfied with using personal phones for professional purposes; they felt that if they were required to do something for their work, their employers should provide the equipment deemed necessary to do it.

The reasons for our hesitance to provide dedicated MOTECH handsets to health facilities were in part financial; using nurses' own phones and relying on SMS would eliminate the upfront cost of hardware provision, thus making the project more accessible to and sustainable for government agencies in resource-limited settings. The SMS versus data issue has been much debated (Donner, 2009). For us, the pivotal point came when we did some calculations around data transmission costs where we found that investing in phones which can transfer information using GPRS actually reduces the total cost of ownership of MOTECH. GPRS data transmission is many times cheaper than SMS. A MOTECH form that requires one to two SMS messages can be transferred in less than 1KB of data, resulting in savings of approximately US $11 per health facility per month[3]. The cost of the dedicated GPRS phone is offset by the savings in data expenditures in just over five months, making the financial sustainability of the project more feasible. Crucially, investing in dedicated MOTECH phones also eliminated our reliance on SMS since Java-enabled phones could be purchased at a low cost. Even low-end Java phones unlocked for us a potential that could not be realized with SMS:

- Firstly, Java-enabled handsets are more suited to poor network areas than SMS because forms can easily be saved on the phone and uploaded when connectivity is restored. We had found network reliability to be a challenge in the rural areas in which we were working, so this was an extremely useful feature.
- Secondly, security features such as user authentication schemes can be built into Java forms, but are not possible with SMS. This is an important aspect of a system that is transferring sensitive patient information.

- Thirdly, leveraging Java-enabled phones from the outset of the program better facilitates the development of more sophisticated applications, without needing to re-train users, re-distribute hardware and softcopy documentation, or change platforms. Therefore, we felt that Java-enabled phones provided a stronger foundation for developing applications, providing more potential for supporting effective service delivery.

We selected the Nokia 1680 for our pilot because it was low cost, had a long battery life, was durable, and 80 per cent of the nurses owned Nokia phones of their own, so we expected them to be more familiar with how to use them than phones from other manufacturers. We issued phones to facilities with an equipment agreement that was developed together with the Ghana Health Service. The agreement indicated that MOTECH handsets should remain in the clinic or any other place of service delivery at all times. It included a penalty for nurses in the case that a phone was lost or stolen owing to negligence. Levying a penalty for a lost or stolen phone is at the discretion of the district director. Therefore, if she or he decides that the phone was lost or stolen not owing to any negligence on the part of the nurse, she or he can decide not to enforce the penalty. We ensured that the penalty was low enough and left enough room for discretion that it would not deter nurses from using the phones. Should the penalty be imposed, it is shared by all the nurses at a facility, with the majority being paid by the nurse who lost the phone. This shared responsibility model was created in order to encourage nurses to accept joint responsibility for the handsets and to support each other in keeping it safe.

Nurse incentivization

We found in situ testing to be extremely important for maximizing the quality of the feedback for system design. We held several workshops in which nurses tried out applications in role play. These were useful for highlighting issues with navigating the application or training challenges, but had limited value for inviting discussion on which additional features would be most useful, how the application would alter or integrate with existing workflow or potential benefits and annoyances of the application in the nurses' daily routine. Therefore, we also requested nurses to use the prototype of the application with real patients in their facilities for one month, as if the service were already live. This enabled nurses to really experience the effect of the application on their work, to the extent that they were able to suggest improvements and new features that they believed would help them. This was invaluable for enabling us to modify existing parts of the application and even spec out new features in direct response to the suggestions of the nurses.

In this prototyping stage, nurses identified that they thought the application would result in time savings and better information flow. They anticipated that time savings would come from the automation of monthly reports. In the design of the system, this was intended to be the main incentive for nurses to enter data into MOTECH. However, when MOTECH was actually implemented, we found that initially nurses did not recognize automated reports as an incentive. In the field, nurses were requesting us to buy lunch for them in return for the extra work MOTECH was making them do, and some even asked for money. We think that this originated from two aspects of how the project was implemented.

- Firstly, the benefits of automated reporting cannot be realized until data is submitted for every single client seen in a month. Unless all data is entered, reports are inaccurate, so nurses are required to add in the data for those clients whose information was not submitted to MOTECH. Therefore, in the ramp-up stage of the project when nurses are becoming used to the application, reports are unlikely to be complete meaning that nurses do not save time on reporting at all. We tried calling nurses to encourage them to enter all forms, and monitored their daily uploads so that we could prompt them when no data had been sent. We set up competitions in which the most active facilities would receive small gifts such as radios. These encouragement methods seemed to be quite effective, and we are seeing successful use of MOTECH in the facilities, with nurses now realizing its benefits. We were surprised by how constant this encouragement needs to be (literally daily), and how time-intensive it is to support this. We have come to realize how using new technology in these setting is a really significant shift in work practices and culture, and so its integration will take time.
- Secondly, MOTECH was seen as a discrete new 'project' by nurses. Instead of seeing MOTECH as an element of their normal responsibilities as Ghana Health Service employees, nurses regarded it as something extra brought to them by an external organization that would one day go away. We think this was because the project timescales meant that we were required to work in facilities testing applications with nurses at the same time as developing the higher level relationship with the Ghana Health Service. Therefore our first interactions with nurses were when the relationship with the Ghana Health Service was in its nascent stages; they could see this and so the project appeared to be coming from an external entity. Therefore, we worked more closely with the Ghana Health Service so that their staff was more *visibly* active in the project and a Technical Working Group was set up to ensure closer liaison

between MOTECH staff and Ghana Health Service staff to ensure seamless coordination in the field, aspects of collaboration which would ideally have been in place from the beginning. These steps improved the nurses' perception of the level of Ghana Health Service ownership of MOTECH, which in turn improved the consistency with which they submitted data, better enabling them to see the benefits of automated reporting.

Community volunteer incentivization

The Ghana Health Service has a system through which each community has health volunteers who are responsible for liaising between health facilities and community members. As part of their Ghana Health Service responsibilities, these volunteers have also become ambassadors for MOTECH. They are tasked with assisting new clients to register into the system, helping existing clients to access their messages and reporting recent unattended child births into the system. When the project was launched, these volunteers were invited for training and issued with T-shirts and promotional flyers and posters. We had heard other projects say that the community status gained from working with projects was a sufficient incentivization to keep volunteers involved. We have found this assertion to be overrated and have found that volunteers seek an opportunity for income generation or rewards such as bikes, radios, and phones. We will soon, therefore, we are currently considering a reward scheme in which airtime units are issued to volunteers per interaction with MOTECH.

Partnerships

Government

Technology organizations typically have a flat organizational structure in which there are few levels between staff and managers, employees of all levels are involved in decision-making processes and there is free communication between junior and senior staff. It follows, then, that Grameen Technology Center follows a similar ethos. Adjusting this working culture for a more hierarchical government structure took time and discipline. Communicating appropriately with government proved critical to the success of our important partnership with the Ghana Health Service. Some learnings in this area include:

- Government needs to be engaged as an equal partner in design, implementation, and oversight, including managing the challenges.
- It is important to follow proper protocol and demonstrate respect for government institutions, culture, and expectations.

- The project needs to directly support national priorities.
- For success the project needs rational endorsement, approval, and leadership from within the government entity.
- The project needs an understanding of the role of national, regional, and district level government and how to engage with them.
- Projects should recognize the need to provide extra functional support to facility the involvement of government at different levels.
- Projects should be aware of different partner organizations working in the same area, to avoid being a coordination burden for the government entity.

Academic institutions

Columbia University is undertaking a social impact assessment of the MOTECH pilot implementation in the Upper East Region in order to determine the impact of the mobile intervention. The challenge with how this and many other grants are set up is that there is very limited time to design and build applications, implement, and prove impact; for MOTECH all this had to be achieved in two years. The difficulty here is that introducing mobile technology to a well-established paper-based manual system introduces a substantial shift and requires workers to adapt long-standing working practices in order to accommodate the intervention. It takes a lot of time, therefore, for the system to stabilize – both technically and operationally – to a point at which it could be considered to be operating smoothly enough for an impact assessment to be conducted. We have had to continuously re-prioritize technical and operational tasks to ensure the rigor of the social impact assessment, and our colleagues at Columbia University have also had to be ready to alter research plans to allow for suitable stabilization of the system. Another challenge with research in short grants is that social impact results, which would make donor proposals more compelling, are not available until after the initial funding ends.

While there is much emphasis on achieving social impact, there are many formative learnings that have a lot of value to the project and potential future implementations; we believe that these should not be overlooked. We have found it to be useful to take some time every few months to think reflexively through what has been learned, what mistakes we would avoid in the future, and which successes we would like to carry forward. Many such learnings and decision points have been explained here, and more can be found in 'MOTECH Ghana: Lessons Learned So Far', available online. We intend that noting these aspects will assist future iterations of the project and will enable other implementers to see the logic behind some of the decisions made.

Telecommunications operators

Establishing infrastructure to enable our software systems to interact with mobile network operators was a much more time-consuming process than we anticipated, an experience shared by other development projects and private sector. Acquiring a short code that could be used across multiple network operators – a valuable revenue generator for telecommunications companies – took twelve months. Installing and configuring E1 lines to connect with all the telecommunications networks took even longer. Projects should get a very early start on building their communication systems with network operators.

Conclusions

MOTECH has taught us much about how to develop applications not only for end-users, but also in organizational settings. As has been explored here, there are common themes to designing applications for these users, as well as some differences. Some of these are explained here:

Table 8.1 Some common themes when designing mobile applications for end-users and organizational settings

Designing for End-Users	Designing for Clinic/Organizational Settings
User-recognized lack of information drives demand for service which is seen as something with potential for personal benefit (being more informed, having better health). This makes the marketing message quite straightforward.	Demand for service comes from organization, which does not always translate into recognition of need for technology intervention by individuals (nurses). Seeing the personal benefit is to some extent dependent on personal satisfaction derived from doing a thorough job, so is not universally present. This presents a challenge to uptake and compliance, and can limit the success of efforts to encourage that.
Necessary to use a technology familiar to the user to enable uptake.	Possible to introduce new technologies owing to greater capacity to train staff.
Intervention works because it slots into the everyday routines of the user. Users typically already use phones, already receive and make calls, etc.	Potential benefit of the intervention lies partly in its change of a process of workflow. This also makes it more difficult to integrate the service into the routines of the health worker than for end-users.

Designing for End-Users	Designing for Clinic/Organizational Settings
No apparent business model which makes provision of mobile phones a viable option, forcing dependency on common channels – voice and SMS.	Total cost of ownership is reduced by providing phones to nurses, enabling use of data and more sophisticated apps.
Credibility through association with respected partners is important for people to trust the information.	Credibility is gained only through demonstrating Ghana Health Service ownership of the intervention.
Critical that intervention is not seen as a standalone effort but one that complements other parallel behavior change initiatives.	Critical that intervention is situated in an existing ecosystem. For instance, phones cannot have an impact unless they are implemented alongside efforts to improve service delivery.

Notes

1 This chapter is a distillation of some of the main themes explored in Grameen Foundation's self-published document 'MOTECH Early Lessons Learned', available at http://www.grameenfoundation.org/sites/default/files/MOTECH-Early-Lessons-Learned-March-2011-FINAL.pdf. While the self-published document is a summary of main learning outcomes and actions taken, this chapter explores in more detail and in a more discursive manner, the processes and methods used in developing the applications with particular attention to client and nurse behavior change. Grameen Foundation permits the release of this shorter document and its inclusion in this publication.

2 In Ghana, the term 'flashing' refers to the act of giving someone a missed call: calling a number for a few seconds and hanging up before the recipient has time to answer. Some studies estimate that flashes make up 20 per cent to 30 per cent of all calls made in Africa.

3 An SMS on MTN, Ghana's leading mobile carrier, costs 0.045 GHS per message. 1 kb of GPRS data costs 0.000195 per kb. On average, CHPS compounds in the KND district send 360 messages per month, based on 2009 DHIMS reports.

References

AudienceScapes (2009), 'National Survey of Ghana', Washington, DC: InterMedia. http://www.audiencescapes.org/africa-research-online-data-analysis-tool-survey-information [Accessed 15 February 2012].

Donner, J. (2009), 'Mobile-Based Livelihood Services in Africa: Pilots and Early Deployments', in M. Fernandez-Ardevol and A. Ros (eds), *Communication Technologies in Latin America and Africa: A Multidisciplinary Perspective*, Barcelona: IN3: 37–58.

Erickson, B., Lind, A., Johnson, B. and O'Barr, W. (1978), 'Speech Style and Impression Formation in a Court Setting: The Effects of "Powerful" and "Powerless" Speech', *Journal of Experimental Social Psychology* 14(3): 266–79.

Fontelo, P., Liu, F., Zhang, K., Ackerman, M. and Tolentino, H. (2008), 'The One Laptop Per Child (OLPC) Computer for Health Clinics in Developing Countries', *AMIA Annual Symposium Proceedings*: 192–6.
Heesacker, M., Petty, R. and Cacioppo, J. (1983), 'Field Dependence and Attitude Change: Source Credibility Can Alter Persuation by Affecting Message-Relevant Thinking', *Journal of Personality* 51(4).
ITU. (2009), 'Measuring the Information Society: The ICT Development Index', http://www.itu.int/pub/D-IND-ICTOI-2009 [Accessed 15 February 2012].
Mechael, P. (2009), Motech mHealth Ethnography Report.
Pornpitakpan, C. (2004), 'The Persuasiveness of Source Credibility: A Critical Review of Five Decades' Evidence', *Journal of Applied Social Psychology* 34(2): 243–81.
Sternthal, B., Dholakia, R. and Leavitt, C. (1978), 'The Persuasive Effect of Source Credibility: Tests of Cognitive Response', *The Journal of Consumer Research* 4(4): 252–60.

9 Experiences from the MediNet Project

The programmer's perspective

Salys Sultan and Permanand Mohan, University of West Indies, Trinidad and Tobago

Project summary

The MediNet Project (Mohan and Sultan, 2009) started back in 2007 as a response to a Microsoft External Research Request for Proposals (Microsoft, 2007). The theme was 'Cell phone as a Platform for Health Care'. The main objective of the project was to develop a Caribbean-wide healthcare management system that would pool the heathcare resources of the Caribbean Islands. The core technology proposed for the design of this integrated system was the mobile phone. In the Caribbean region, mobile ownership surpasses computer ownership and landline service (Galperin and Mariscal, 2007). This is primarily due to the lower cost associated with acquiring the devices and the fact that the introduction of wireless telecommunication has made it possible to reach areas that were previously disconnected.

The first phase of the project was the design and development of a *remote patient monitoring system* for Trinidad and Tobago. For this pilot study, the diseases initially targeted were diabetes and cardiovascular disease, two diseases with a high prevalence in the region, but the system was designed to scale to meet the needs of other chronic diseases such as asthma and cancer.

The MediNet architecture is broken down into three main components: the patient interface, a collection of healthcare web services, and the healthcare provider interface. The patient interface comprises a mobile phone and the patients' physiological meters (glucometer and blood pressure meter). The patients use their mobile phone to record their health data. Recordings include their blood sugar reading, their blood pressure reading, their food intake, and daily exercise. The readings from the physiological meters are automatically transferred to the phone using Bluetooth technology. The mobile phone has a software application called 'My Daily Record' that acts as an electronic diary for the recording of the patient's health data. The application allows the patient to enter the readings, view past readings, and enter information regarding their caloric intake and the amount of time spent exercising. The application has a *view tip* feature that allows the patient to receive feedback on the most recent recordings made. This type of feedback is personalized, because it is tailored to the individual patient's current status as opposed to a *one-size-fits-all* approach.

The next component of the MediNet system is a collection of healthcare web services. This component is the mechanism that orchestrates the receipt of data (recordings) from the distributed mobile phone units, as well as delivery of data (feedback to patients, reminders to patients, and alerts to healthcare providers) to the devices. The data transfer takes place using GPRS over a GSM network. These web services are made available through a remote server. This server acts as a central repository for the patient healthcare data. A subset of this data is also stored on the mobile device so that the patients can access their data even without reception. Data on the phone and on the server are encrypted, and a protocol was designed to ensure the integrity of data when it is received at the destination point.

The healthcare provider's interface acts as a portal to the patients' healthcare data. The healthcare provider can monitor their patients' health status remotely and provide feedback when exceptional cases occur. In these cases, alerts are sent to the healthcare provider's mobile phone. The portal provides different views on the patients' data set. The current implementation of the portal takes the form of a website which a doctor or caregiver can access using a computer.

How we got started

The MediNet project (short for Medical Networks) came out of a request for proposals from Microsoft External Research. The theme for that year was the use of cellphones as a platform for healthcare. The call sought 'to incubate creative and novel healthcare solutions that are accessible, affordable, and relevant for "smart" mobile phones. An additional focus was the creation of appropriate services, systems, and infrastructures to provide solutions to the global healthcare community' (Microsoft, 2007). Kristin Tolle, the director of program management at Microsoft External Research, was our main point of contact and overseer for our project.

This was our first experience with a mobile health initiative. To kick-off the project, a group of researchers at the University of the West Indies, including myself, brainstormed on the different ways that the cellphone could be used to provide healthcare services. The main issue that arose was the challenges faced in the Caribbean region when it came to the management of chronic noncommunicable diseases (CNCDs) – one of the main causes of deaths (Douglas 2007). From the beginning, we decided to keep the focus on two diseases – diabetes and cardiovascular disease, but always keeping in mind how the system would be able to scale to support other diseases.

In his book, *Development as Freedom*, Amartya Sen warns of the tendency to identify human capacities with human capital. Human capital considerations focus on the human capacity to augment production possibilities. In contrast, Sen advocates that human capacities should focus on the ability (or substantive freedom) of people '... to lead the lives they have reason to value and to enhance the real choices they have' (Sen, 1999). A range of freedoms is then presented as the foundation of the Good Life; these freedoms are the means by which wealth is generated or the ends which become a more effective means to economic ends. It should be noted that diabetes and other CNCDs are lifestyle diseases and control can be achieved through behavior modification. Taking Sen's line of reasoning, a substantive freedom of diabetics and persons suffering from CNCDs is to take better care of themselves causing them to lead the lives they have reason to value. This freedom will ultimately result in more productive lives and less impact on the economy. Clearly then, tackling diabetes and other CNCDs through behavior modification can play a significant role in developing countries (Sen, 1999).

Our vision took into account this notion of freedom. We saw the patient's mobile phone as a tool to collect medical data within the patient's home or work environment, and allow the patient to make more informed decisions regarding his health. Each patient's medical history would then be stored electronically and compared to the data originating from the patient's cellular phone. Based on the data collected, the system would recommend a certain course of action to be taken by the patient or may notify other agencies, depending on the severity of the case. This would result in better diagnosis, prevention, and routine health management. By implementing the system across the Caribbean region, a distributed system would be obtained where most of the knowledge concerning diseases can be shared among countries. It was noted that most of the healthcare services that may be available to a patient are likely to be in the same country, so it would be necessary to create countrywide networks (called MediNets) that would connect to the overall healthcare management system. The originally proposed architecture of each MediNet is shown in Figure 9.1. It focused primarily on cardiovascular disease and diabetes but can be extended to other medical diseases in later phases.

This vision came from the fact that there was a need to increase the availability of healthcare services in the Caribbean region and the mobile phone was seen as a platform with the potential for great impact. Mobile phones are widespread in the Caribbean with some people even owning two. We were proposing that the mobile

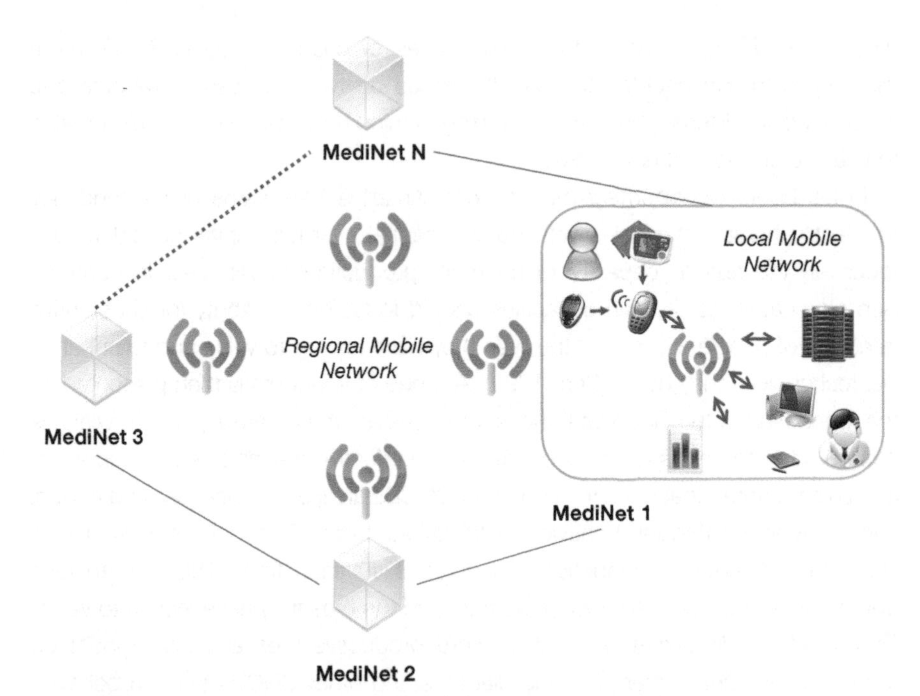

Figure 9.1 Architecture of proposed MediNet

phone act as an 'electronic log' to mirror the daily recording process that was required by diabetics. The connectivity offered by the device afforded the exchange of health data, so once the phone was connected to a telecommunications network, data captured and stored locally could be transmitted to remote areas such as the healthcare provider's location. This was seen as 1) increasing the reach of the services offered and 2) allowing shifting the management of the disease from the healthcare provider to the patient.

The project team was mostly composed of students, researchers, and lecturers in the Department of Computing and Information Technology at the University of the West Indies, St Augustine campus, Trinidad and Tobago. Each member was assigned a role. Dr Permanand Mohan was the principal investigator, and Salys Sultan was the project manager and lead system developer. There were five software engineers, Dylan Marin, Adil Sheikh, Kris Manohar, Phaedra Mohammed and Akash Harriram. Since we were all computer scientists, we brought onboard Dr Ahad Deen, a medical doctor who worked with diabetic patients. The first task that we addressed was getting a better understanding of the current healthcare problem and challenges faced by both doctors and patients – two of the primary users of the system.

Our investigations

One of the main challenges faced by the Caribbean population was that of accessibility to healthcare services (Fraser, 2001). Presently, patients only see their healthcare provider, once or twice in a year and diabetes-related information is not as readily available. Patients also kept poor records of their health status, so consultations with their doctor were left to memory recollection. Another major challenge was cost, that is, costs associated with the care of diabetes and its related complications. We saw prevention as the key to minimizing these costs. Given our technical background, there was a need to investigate further the leading causal agents for these challenges.

We followed a user-centered design methodology (Norman, 1988). This methodology was selected given the fact that mHealth on a whole was new to the Caribbean region and the target user group would not be familiar with *what to expect* from it. We believed once we got the users of the system involved from the early stages and throughout the system design, there was a higher probability that the final system would meet the needs of various stakeholders. We met with professionals in the field, medical students, and, of course, patients. This project had a personal slant to it, as a member of the team had some family members who have been living with diabetes, some even bed-ridden due to complications resulting from the disease. These meetings allowed us to get a better and clearer picture on 'how things were currently done'. It was important to get all the key stakeholders involved from the start so as to design and develop a system that meets the needs of its users, as well as, to design a system that complemented/augmented the current rituals of the target users.

From these interviews, we were able to understand the gaps present in the healthcare system and identify how information and telecommunications technology (ICT) can be harnessed to fill some of these gaps. It was also important for us to establish from the start that we did not see the use of ICT as a replacement of a doctor, nurse, or healthcare provider but more of a way of extending the reach of healthcare, as well as engaging the patient more in the self-care process. We recognized that a healthcare system of this nature had to be more patient-centric than provider-centric, since the treatment of chronic diseases requires a preventative care model.

As a technical person, it was also important for us to know more about the disease itself. As we mentioned before, some family members have been living with this disease, so we had some basic understanding but a deeper understanding was required, especially in the area of prevention. In order to design a system that was effective, there was a need to understand the nature of the disease. We turned to the existing literature in search of current standards and practices.

One of the first articles we came across was the *National Standards for Diabetes Self-Management Education* (Funnell, Brown, Childs, Haas, Hosey, Jensen, Marynink, Peyrot, Piette, Reader, Siminerio, Weinger, and Weiss, 2008). The article provided guidelines on how to approach a DSME initiative including a defined curriculum on what content areas a diabetic should concentrate. This became the foundation for the educational component of the system.

One of the main objectives of the system was to improve the self-management practices of patients. This required a change management model. Human beings are creatures of habit and routine. The problem with most efforts at change is that the conscious effort cannot be sustained over the long term. Therefore, for a new mobile health initiative to be sustained, it is important to build engagement (Sultan, Mohan and Sultan, 2009). Engagement is the skillful mobilization of the energy required to achieve extraordinary results in any mission that really matters. This occurs when people are 'physically energized, emotionally connected, mentally focused and spiritually aligned' (Loehr and Schwartz, 2003). The *LGE Keys* provides three steps involved in building engagement:

1. Facing the truth
2. Defining purpose
3. Taking action

In the first step, the patient must face the truth and acknowledge that healthcare is important and required; this is the key motivating factor. The next step involves determining what needs to be done to achieve the desired state. In this context, it will involve improved self-management and overall well-being. Lastly, the third step is the conversion of the plan into action or doing what is required to achieve the desired objectives. Here is where mobile technology can have the greatest impact.

We incorporated these three steps in the design of the patient interface. The main thrust is that in order for a new ritual to develop, a minimum of thirty to sixty days was required of conscious effort before the new ritual turns into a habit. A ritual in this context is defined as a consciously acquired habitual pattern of thinking and acting that leads to a desired state. The key was to install good practices in the patient's life through the creation of rituals. Examples could include introducing exercise into his life, changing eating habits, or breaking a smoking habit. It is in this process of ritual building that the mobile phone made a positive impact. Since the patients used their mobile devices on a daily basis, we expected them to now use the health application regularly so as to develop a new habit.

We also used some works out of the Center for Creative Leadership (CCL). The CCL has developed a framework for coaching that is supported by a well-tested model of leader development (Ting and Scisco, 2006). This model is built on five areas: the context in which the coaching occurs, assessment, challenge, support, and results. The framework uses coaching as one, but not the only way, to facilitate learning. When coaching is incorporated into a person's day-to-day activities, it becomes a powerful tool which helps people to access and use their lessons of experience.

In the case of eHealth initiatives, the context will depend on ICT that is being employed. For example, in the case of a mobile telemedicine system, the context will be the mobile phone, the device through which the coaching occurs. Therefore, factors such as location, connectivity, the device's screen size, data entry method, and environmental elements that may distract the user's attention must be taken into consideration.

Assessment deals with the unfreezing of present perceptions, providing realistic benchmarks, and understanding developmental needs and the current state of the patient. ICT initiatives which take into account knowledge of the patient and which can tailor the healthcare delivery to meet the patient's individual needs have a greater chance of success.

The healthcare initiative must also challenge the patient by providing an improved pathway to the desired state. Learning is a crucial step in the actualization of the desired state. Therefore, a clear road map on how this can be accomplished is required. Support is also important, as it creates safety for taking risks, ensures that motivation is maintained, and provides the resources necessary for success. Support can come in many forms, for example, by means of a person in the patient's environment, by making available information relating to the patient's illness, and by providing feedback on the patient's current status. Lastly, the results refer to the direct and indirect outcomes – a desired state with lasting impact. In the context of patient-oriented e-health initiative, the desired result is often the patient being in an improved state of health.

Change is difficult. Human beings are creatures of habit and routine; what we did yesterday is what we are likely to do today. The problem with most efforts at change is that conscious effort cannot be sustained over the long term. Will and discipline are far more limited resources than most people recognize. When developing new rituals, it is necessary to be as precise as possible in both the timing and behavior to habitualize, as well as focus on acquiring only a few major rituals at any one time. Moreover, it is important to create an environment that is supportive during the ritual acquisition period. In the healthcare context, it is expected that a doctor or caregiver will work with the patient on the development of the new ritual. This should result in an improvement plan consisting of new habits and routines, thereby reducing the dependence on conscious self-regulated behaviors.

In the first step, the patient must first face the truth and acknowledge that the self-care is important and required. The next step involves determining what needs to be done to achieve the desired state (i.e. improved self-management and overall well-being). The third step is the conversion of the plan into action or doing what is required to achieve the desired objectives. These three steps nurture the ritual building process and it is this area where ICT initiatives can make the biggest impact on the healthcare domain.

Applying computer science to health

Once we had a clear understanding of the existing problem and the challenges associated with current ways of doing things, the next step was to identify possible solutions to address these challenges. The mobile phone was seen as a suitable platform to address some of these challenges. In the Caribbean region, mobile phones usage is very high. Most people owned one or even two mobile phones and this is mainly because the cost of owning a mobile phone is low and the wireless communication has enabled communication to some previously disconnected areas. The mobile phone also allows for a one-on-one mapping with patient and phone. It is a personal device; therefore, services offered through the phone can be tailored to the patient. This was one of the objectives of the study – to deliver personalized healthcare services through the mobile phone.

The MediNet project brought together skills from different areas in computer science (CS): mobile applications development, database design, user interface design, and web programming to name a few. Given that the choice of platform was the mobile phone, new skills were required in application development on small devices which had some physical constraints. At the start of the project and as part of the Microsoft awarded grant, we were provided with some HTC smartphones running Mobile Windows 6.0 Professional. This was our programming platform which was new frontier for the project team. In the next subsections, we explore some of the notable aspects of designing, developing, and implementing a mobile health solution.

Communication protocols

One of the features of the proposed system was to allow the patient to capture/log their daily readings. We were interested in how this could be done automatically without too much intervention by the patient. To achieve this, we needed the appropriate communication libraries to enable the exchange of data between the phone and the respective physiological meter (Sultan and Mohan, 2009). Our research showed that there were three popular communication protocols with existing healthcare systems: USB, RS-232, and Bluetooth. Some vendors of healthcare meters provide USB port on their healthcare meters. These USB ports offer slave connectivity. This made them only compatible with a PC USB port. Therefore, USB-enabled healthcare monitors were not suitable for healthcare monitoring systems that use a mobile phone as the data access point.

Hardware implementation of RS-232 was simple; therefore, some vendors provided RS-232 connectivity with their healthcare meters. However, mobile phones available in the market do not contain RS-232 ports. Therefore, this option was not suitable for healthcare monitoring systems based on mobile telephony. Being a short-range and low-power communication protocol, Bluetooth was being used by some vendors of healthcare meters for communication between the monitors and PC or mobile phone.

Since Bluetooth was also very popular in mobile phone communication, it became an ideal candidate for transferring readings from the healthcare monitor to the mobile phone. Moreover, Bluetooth has been proven to have high data transfer rates, surpassing serial and parallel ports. Therefore, in our research, we only examined healthcare systems that used the Bluetooth protocol for communication between the mobile phone and the measuring devices. We narrowed down our selection to three Bluetooth enabled glucometer devices, then we chose the one that had an open programmable interface. At the time of this project, there was only one Bluetooth-enabled blood pressure meter available on the market.

It is important to note that there was no established mobile-to-healthcare meter communication standard; therefore, customization was required for each type of physiological device used. For our study, we used a LifeScan One Touch glucometer and an A&D Blood Pressure meter, both using the Bluetooth protocol to transfer results. In the case of the glucometer, additional accessory created by the PolyMap company was also needed to enable the Bluetooth transmission. At the beginning of the project, it was our intention to minimize the amount of data the user had to enter manually, that is why we used meters with some form of communication protocol. The assumption was the less input required by the user will make the data entry task easier to perform. However, after user trials, the communication problems that prevailed due to the use of the Bluetooth technology outweighed this perceived benefit. These communication problems are discussed in the 'Lessons Learned' section and the user trials are discussed in the 'Testing and Evaluation' section.

Data storage

For data storage and sharing, we designed a database that was hosted on a remote server. At the time of this research, online electronic health records (EHR) systems such as MS Health Vault and Google Health were not available, so we developed our own custom EHR referred to as the *patient record*. This record held demographic information on the patient as well as the daily readings that were logged by the user. A subset of the patient record was stored on the patient's mobile phone. This was to ensure that the user had access to information even if they were not connected to the telecommunications network. Therefore, protocols were developed to ensure that the data stored on the local store and on the remote data store were in sync.

One of the interesting and more cost-effective features of the mobile application was that it allowed multiple users from the same family to access the system in a seamless manner. This entailed having a logon feature and also keeping different data sets for each member of the family. This was successfully tested in the trial by granting a patient's husband access to the system; he used the same blood pressure meter and blood glucose meter to take his readings.

Data integrity

One notable programming task when it came to applications of this nature was the 'seriousness of purpose'. When dealing with healthcare applications, the data captured and the results being processed and transferred can mean the difference between life and death; therefore, the integrity of the data stored and transferred was of paramount importance. Furthermore, the personal nature of health information means that data privacy and data protection are required. We had to address the fact that we were relying on a mobile telecommunications network to transfer data, and this network may not be reliable (i.e. the network might be 'down' or data packets sent may be dropped/lost). To ensure the integrity of data, custom protocols and algorithms were used to ensure that the data transferred was in fact the data received. Encryption algorithms were used to secure the data, on the local store, during the transmission, and on the remote store.

Usability

Another CS skill required was the design of the user interface. The two main interfaces for this system were the Patient Interface and the Health Care Provider Portal as shown in Figure 9.2. The Patients Interface included the mobile phone, the application running on the mobile phone, and the patient's physiological meters. The Health Care Provider interface included a web portal that was accessed through a computer.

When designing the interfaces for the patient and doctor, we used paper prototyping. Some mock screens were drafted and focus groups were conducted to elicit feedback on the usability of the interfaces. Given the small screen size of the mobile phone and the fact that one of the complications relating to diabetes is

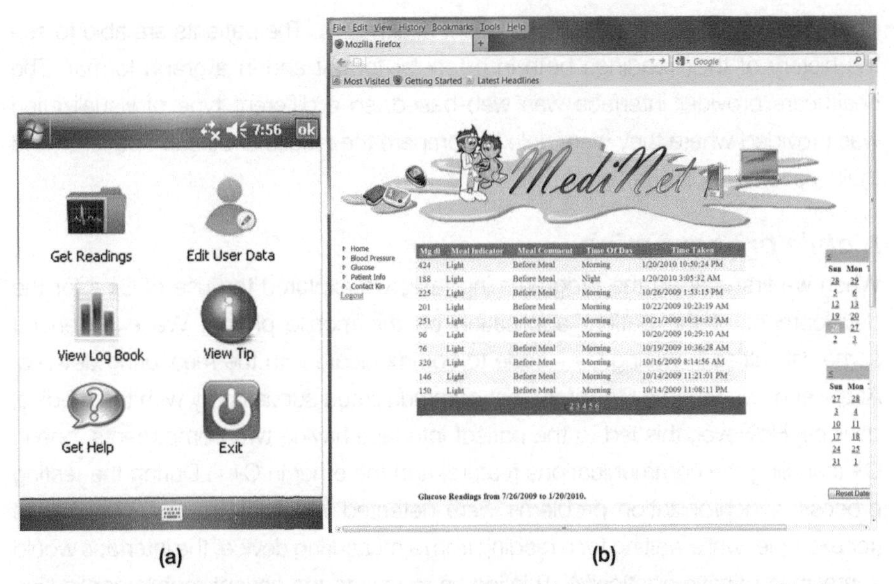

Figure 9.2 User interfaces: (a) patient interface and (b) healthcare providers interface

impaired vision, special considerations are needed to address these challenges. For example, the maximum font size allowable may still be too small, especially for a diabetic with eye problems. We plan to address these issues in the next version of the application by incorporating appropriate graphical symbols and audio.

For the selection of mobile phone for the patient, a focus group was conducted to obtain some preliminary feedback on the current mobile phone usage within the target user group and the impressions on different models of mobile phones. The patients were presented with two types of phones: a Windows-based smartphone that was controlled through stylus-input and a Java-based phone with keypad user entry. The users were asked to complete defined tasks on the different phones and the time taken to complete each task, along with the users' feedback, were recorded. Overall, the users preferred the use of the smartphone (including some users who were not expert phone users) because of the perceived ease of data entry and the graphical user interface capabilities provided. A study was also performed on the usability of the glucometer and blood pressure meter that were selected for use in the MediNet project. It was important that the users felt comfortable with each component of the system.

From our study, it was evident that the mobile phone presented many constraints in terms of user interaction and device processing capabilities. The limited screen size meant that data input was restricted to a small onscreen keypad. This was also another motivation behind the automatic data transfer. We also wanted to create different data visualizations for the patient health data. The patients are able to see the history of their readings both in a tabular format and in a graph format. The healthcare provider interface was web-based, so a different type of visualization was provided where they were able to compare the results of different patients and their associative parameters.

Mobile programming

When we first started the programming task, we explored the use of C++ for the development of the patient application on the mobile phone. We experienced some difficulties in writing C++ code to communicate with the measuring devices. At the end, we found a C# library that communicated successfully with the medical devices. However, this led to the patient interface having two components, one in C# (handling the communications feature) and the other in C++. During the testing process, synchronization problems were detected which caused usability issues (for example, while waiting for a reading from a measuring device, the interface would sometimes behave erratically). This led us to rewrite the patient mobile application in C# so that there was no need to synchronize two independent programs on the mobile phone. We also decided to go with C# as the language for a full scale mobile application versus another language for a web-based application because a reliable internet access was not always available.

Limited memory on the phone is also a challenge when it came to mobile programming. We tried to store only frequently accessed data on the phone. For example, in the case of the patient's history of readings, we stored about 100 days of readings on the phone itself. This was acceptable for the first version but in a later version we are planning to generate reports spanning longer periods at the server which are downloaded on request by the mobile device to display to the patient.

When it came to the patient feedback mechanism as programmers we were inclined to code the system using a rules-based approach but that was a challenge given the very nature of healthcare – i.e. what might work for one patient may not be the same for another. For example, a 'good' blood sugar reading for one patient may be seen as a high reading for another. Each patient is different and therefore personalized and adaptive systems are needed to meet the individual needs of each patient.

Testing and evaluation

Fifteen Type 2 diabetic patients were recruited from the doctor's practice to participate in a six-month field trial (July 2009 to December 2009). The participation was on a voluntary basis. To prepare each phone for the trial, we installed the mobile application and tested each device to ensure it worked as expected. We created log in credentials for each patient and healthcare provider.

For the first meeting with the patients, we executed two questionnaires: a patient profile questionnaire, to capture demographic data as well as current healthcare practices and a mobile usage questionnaire to gage how the patient presently used their mobile devices. A demonstration of the system was then conducted. It is at this demonstration we experienced first hand the problems inherent with the wireless communication between the mobile phone and the physiological meters. It is worth noting that we gave the demonstration at a clinic which had many types of equipment communicating at differing frequencies. We came to the conclusion that the wireless transmission failed because of the interference by other devices.

The patients were allowed to use the system in their home or work environment. Each patient was given a glucometer, blood pressure meter, and a mobile phone running the patient interface software. Because of the C++ and C# synchronization problems, the patients complained of usability issues but after the fully C# application was installed in September 2009, there were no further issues of this nature.

The doctor was also trained on the use of the Health Care Providers portal, and he monitored his patients remotely for the six-month period. During this period, he provided feedback via SMS and phone calls to his patients. Table 9.1 summarizes the feedback obtained from the patients after the first two months of the field study, for more discussion this feedback, see Sultan and Mohan (in press).

Table 9.1 Field study results

Feature	**Value**
Type of diabetes	Type 2
Participation Count (end of trial)	7
Residence	Trinidad and Tobago
Most popular day of usage	Mondays
Time taken to get comfortable with system	10–15 days
Ranking of most used featured of app	Get Readings, View Log, View Tip
Groups overall compliance	70%
Preferred history of readings view	Tabular
Users satisfied with system	100%
Users who will recommend system to family or friend	100%

Lessons learned

The project team combined had over fifteen years of programming experience in both academia and the industry, but this was our first experience with a health system. There were many lessons learned from this mobile health initiative. A deeper awareness and understanding of the issues faced by regular citizens of the Caribbean region in obtaining quality (if at all, any) healthcare services and the important role that mobile technology can play in providing healthcare services at a cheaper cost. An understanding of how software components can be developed to tackle many of the problems that plague healthcare systems in the region and an understanding of how software technologies commonly used today (for example Facebook-like systems) can be used to support the healthcare system. This is actually a spin-off of the MediNet project, another project called Mobile DSMS concentrates on the formation of virtual peer support groups using mobile phones.

Before the MediNet project, our programming focus or scope was narrow within a particular organization, discipline, and/or programming task. The MediNet project has incorporated a wide cross section within the computer science field as well as an integration with medical and behavioral sciences. We have a greater appreciation of the many factors involved in the design, implementation, and introduction of a new mobile health initiative as well as the realities involved with field work. In the medical space, our knowledge of the disease itself has increased and particularly in different ways, technology can be used in the disease management process. As mentioned before, in terms of behavioral science scope, we involved an external consultant who specialized in coaching initiatives targeted toward behavior change. This was addressed early on in the design stage because the proposed system was intended to in fact effect change. Working in these different disciplines meant that we had to be open to the reality of how current systems and practices worked and be creative in the application of ICT to effect behavior change. The consultant played an important role in explaining how the behavior theory was applied to different change management contexts, as well as providing feedback throughout our design, development, and testing phases. At times in our conversations, we had to make sure that we all spoke the same language because on the one hand we were dealing with theoretical subject matter and at other times technical implementation details. We now see ourselves as interdisciplinary researchers, always exploring ways in which the intersection of various disciplines can be used to generate new possibilities in the area of disease management.

Given our background, our contributions to mobile health included the ability to transform user and system requirements into a fully tested working system.

An understanding of user-centered design and the prototyping process: the importance of considering the user during the design process (for example in designing the user interface), implementation, and evaluation stages. We also have a keen awareness and understanding of the problems faced by the target audience as well as the unmet needs because of first-hand experience with a person belonging to the target audience. Our skills in teamwork helped keep the project team focused. We met regularly and worked together to iron out issues that were new to the area of mobile health, for example, how to treat with the sensitivity of the data being stored and transferred using a third-party telecommunications network, and the protocols used to transfer data between the mobile phone and the physiological meters. We also ensured that each of the technical challenges faced (the availability and reliability of telecommunications network, the design of a user interface on a small screen size with limited keyboard features, communication interferences using a wireless communication protocol, and the limited processing capabilities of the mobile phone) were addressed in a seamless fashion so as to not disrupt the user's experience.

Conclusion

Words of advice to other programmers entering this domain: the health space provides enormous potential for the development of software technology which can enable the provision of many unique forms of healthcare services (this can be very rewarding when one looks at the lives that are saved/improved due to the use of a system). However, the intended users of the software must always be considered in the development process, and user interfaces should be designed as simply as possible. Systems should concentrate on the value that intended users will gain from using the system rather than having impressive hard-to-use features which are seldom used. It is also important to become familiar with healthcare standards/ government regulations and understand the implications of these standards/ regulations on software being developed. Many different software development skills are required depending on the available resources and target delivery platform, and programmers would need to develop expertise in many of them. Teamwork is also very important, given the many facets of software development associated with a healthcare system and the different stakeholders involved.

References

Fraser, H. (2001), 'The Dilemma of Diabetes: Health Care Crisis in the Caribbean', *Revista Panamericana de Salud Publica* 9(2): 61–4.

Funnell, M., Brown, T., Childs, B., Haas, L., Hosey, G., Jensen, B., Maryniuk, M., Peyrot, M., Piette, J., Reader, D., Siminerio, L., Weinger, K. and Weiss, M. (2008), 'National Standards for Diabetes Self-Management Education', *Diabetes Care* 31 (Supplement 1): S97–S104.

Galperin, H. and Mariscal, J. (2007), 'Mobile Opportunities: Poverty and Mobile Telephony in Latin America and the Caribbean', DIRSI. http://www.dirsi.net/files/regional/REGIONAL_FINAL_english.pdf [Accessed 15 February 2012].

Loehr, J. and Schwartz, T. (2003), *The Power of Full Engagement: Managing Energy, Not Time, Is the Key to High Performance and Personal Renewal*, New York: Free Press.

Microsoft. (2007), 'RFP: Cell Phones as a Platform for Healthcare', http://www.rfpdb.com/view/document/id/1978 [Accessed 21 February 2012].

Mohan, P. and Sultan, S. (2009), *Medinet: A Mobile Healthcare Management System for the Caribbean Region*. 6th Annual International Conference on Mobile and Ubiquitous Systems: Computing, Networking and Services, Toronto, Ontario, Canada.

Norman, D. (1988), *The Design of Everyday Things*, New York: Basic Books.

Sen, A. (1999), *Development as Freedom*, Oxford: Oxford University Press.

Sultan, S. and Mohan, P. (2009), *How to Interact: Evaluating the Interface between Mobile Healthcare Systems and the Monitoring of Blood Sugar and Blood Pressure*. Workshop on Ubiquitous Mobile Healthcare Applications, Toronto, Ontario, Canada.

Sultan, S. and Mohan, P. (in press), 'Transforming Usage Data into a Sustainable Mobile Health Solution', *Electronic Markets - The International Journal on Networked Business*.

Sultan, S., Mohan, P. and Sultan, N. (2009), *Managing Change: Experiences from a New E-Health Initiative for Patients with Diabetes and Cardiovascular Disease*. 1st IEEE International WoWMoM Workshop on Interdisciplinary Research on E-Health Services and Systems, Kos, Greece.

Ting, S. and Scisco, P. (2006), *The Ccl Handbook of Coaching: A Guide for the Leader Coach*, San Francisco: Jossey-Bass.

10 Text to Change

Pioneers in using mobile phones as persuasive technology on health in Africa

Hajo van Beijma and Bas Hoefman, Text to Change

Text to Change

Over the last decade, the mobile technology landscape has changed dramatically across Africa and the developing world. As the solitary most transformative technology for development, mobile phones have ignited economic growth and development; and they have become increasingly affordable and accessible – even to the world's poorest. Mobile subscriptions as by 2010 totaled over 5.3 billion worldwide, and access to mobile networks is now available to 90 per cent of the world's population, with at least over 1 billion mobile subscribers across Africa (Orth, 2011). Explosive growth in the mobile sector had meant that, by early 2007, mobile users constituted almost 90 per cent of all African telephone subscribers. At the end of 2007, there were 280.7 million mobile phone subscribers in Africa, representing a penetration rate of 30.4 per cent (McNamara, 2007).

Inspired by an eye opening Celtel Documentary, aired on BBC News Channel, that highlighted the significant growth of the mobile industry in Africa way back in 2007, Mr Bas Hoefman realized the potential to communicate health information to people via a mobile phone. For a while he nursed this thrilling innovation, considering that his employment at ING Bank, where he had currently been working for two years, was unsatisfactory. Bas therefore encouraged himself to explore this new channel of his career, inspired by an inner drive of faith and hope. Over a few drinks with his friend Hajo van Beijma, with whom he has founded Text to Change (TTC), Bas Hoefman shared his remarkable idea. The proposed solution was to take advantage of the boom in mobile telephony in Africa, using the short message service (SMS) as an easy, cost-effective and interactive way to communicate information, collect data, and create awareness on health issues.

After a challenging start and several unsuccessful grant applications, Bas and Hajo were introduced to Merck & Co, an American pharmaceutical company. Their company foundation was keen to fund innovative ideas and had an affiliate in Uganda (Philips Pharmaceuticals) willing to work with them. Finally, in 2007, the TTC Foundation was born and since then, the combined energy and dedication of the duo has brought TTC well and truly to life.

Starting small: the pilot phase

Research carried out by the Uganda Demographic and Health Survey (UDHS) in 2006 showed that only 30 per cent of women and 40 per cent of men had any comprehensive knowledge of HIV/AIDS. It also revealed that only 71 per cent of women and 77 per cent of men had ever been tested for the disease (Uganda Bureau of Statistics, 2006). With this kind of research proving that HIV/AIDs was a rampant scourge that was eroding Uganda's population, Hajo and Bas thought that the use of mobile phones would then act as a channel to remind people about clinic appointments, taking their medicine and more so, share pertinent information on how to curb the disease.

Also with the rapid growth of mobile phone subscribers in Uganda (approximately 8.2 million in 2008), TTC immediately saw this as an opportunity to reach a large number of people on the HIV/AIDS issue and set about preparing their first pilot project (ITU, 2009). So, in August 2008, the two Text to Change (TTC) founders, together with Marieke Hoefman, a doctor specializing in tropical medicine, flew to Uganda. The trio met with NGOs focusing on HIV prevention campaigns, as well as Celtel Uganda (now known as Airtel Bharti Uganda, formerly known as Zain Uganda, which was one of the dominant Mobile Telecom Operators in Uganda in 2008), who was the telecom provider that was willing to provide text messages (SMS) at a reduced rate.

After numerous Google searches, Bas was surprised that there were not many (large scale) initiatives as he had envisaged, and so he realized the project's potential. He conducted more detailed research through various media such as the internet and local newspapers on several NGOs addressing the HIV/AIDS scourge in Uganda. The determined team identified AIDS Information Centre (AIC), a local NGO, as a potential partner with whom they could establish a pilot project. It was clear through research and subsequent meetings with the partner and the team that AIC had goals to meet with which they were keen to try out new technologies, among these a mobile phone. These goals included:

1. To improve knowledge and awareness about HIV/AIDS in Uganda.
2. To increase the uptake in HIV Voluntary Counseling and Testing (HCT) in their branches throughout Uganda.

Developing the SMS campaign

The team was to reach at least 15,000 mobile phone users (which was the number of mobile numbers AIC had in the database), in AIC's Mbarara region (southwest Uganda) with an interactive SMS campaign to run for six weeks under the slogan '*Don't guess the answers, learn the truth about AIDS*'. We wanted to reach as many people as possible, without being too intrusive with the messaging.

The use of SMS to influence health behavioral change was a novel opportunity that had not been fully explored in Uganda as yet in 2007. Neighboring countries like Kenya have used this approach and can testify that behavior change was triggered by SMS messages among people living with HIV who were taking anti-retroviral medication for HIV (Hahn, 2011). Furthermore, we wanted to capture HIV/AIDS behavioral change data impacted by the use of SMS that would be used for future analysis and research. Therefore, we set up an interactive SMS quiz to test people on their HIV/AIDS knowledge. Participants would receive multiple-choice questions via their mobile phone as well as messages encouraging them to go for testing. Some of the questions were designed to spark discussions on (often) tabooed subjects, such as condom use.

Sample Question:

1. Do you think a healthy looking person could have HIV?
   - a)Yes
   - b)No

Correct reply: Yes! You cannot tell from someone's appearance whether he has HIV or not. You only know by taking an HIV test. So do the test
Wrong reply: Wrong! A healthy looking person can certainly have HIV. You only know by taking an HIV test. So do the test at AIC Arua and know your HIV

Figure 10.1 Sample SMS quiz question

Quote from one of the participants:
"This is exactly the desired open discussion on HIV/AIDS which is needed to reduce stigma."

Figure 10.2 Quote from a participant

Answer sent back by the participants were immediately followed up with an automated response – a confirmation or a rectification. As a further motivator, the quiz also offered a range of prizes, including free airtime and mobile phones.

The idea of using a quiz developed from the fact that traditional health communication campaigns that had been previously carried out by AIC included radio, television, and print media were all a one-way message with the end-user. We believed that SMS quizzes could provide the perfect channel to directly and timely communicate with their target audience who include especially the youths and all Ugandan citizens and could also be a suitable medium to make existing campaigns interactive. For maximum effect, SMS quizzes work best as part of a package of health communication activities enhancing and supporting traditional communication channels such as radio and posters. Not only will you embed your mobile short code in your marketing materials (on billboards, posters, your website, radio, TV, etc.), but you will decide what confirmation message to send back to people texting in, what frequency you will use to send mobile campaign updates and also build a database that can be used for data collection (Calder Strategies, 2007).

The campaign's primary goal was to demonstrate that mobile phones could be a highly effective tool in creating awareness on health topics in developing countries. We had a 20 per cent response rate on the questions, but more importantly, the demand for HCT services at the AIC in Mbarara rose over 40 per cent during the pilot. In total, 255 participants came for HCT services (183 males and 72 females), which represented a 40 per cent increase (ITU, 2010). In general, the participants were reminded about HIV/AIDS and the need to know one's status. They passed the information they gained onto relatives, friends, and others in the community. The participants were informed of different places where they could access HCT services, and TTC realized the cost-effectiveness and convenience of communication via SMS.

The proof of concept that SMS is a simple and very successful way to transfer health information for the interest and needs of target populations and to increase the uptake in health services was evidence enough for us to continue our work.

Growing from the pilot phase

When we look back, finding support for this initiative was a complex start. Convincing firms and organizations to buy in to this new innovation was also difficult. We arranged several meetings with organizations in Uganda, among these were Air Uganda, Nile Breweries, Unilever, and also the AIC. The idea was exciting for the partners, especially in using mobile to market their activities and products, alongside sharing pertinent health information with their clients but also staff members. Many partners were receptive about the idea. The duo was hopeful; however, the partners were always ambiguous and nonresponsive.

But a ray of hope beamed their way, when Merck & Co, an American pharmaceutical company, committed a grant of US $37,500 which was used to work with then Celtel's (now Airtel's) existing text messaging software (designing our own software was too expensive for us at this stage), to launch a marketing campaign for the project and a contribution toward AIC's role. All TTC staff worked voluntarily.

After this initial successful program, we decided to share our experiences with the previous partners we had visited. Reports, white papers, blog posts, website publications, and other material were shared including local news print (Kasozi and Basudde, 2008; Nafula, 2008; Royal Tropical Institute, 2010; TTC, 2010). This opened new doors and opportunities for funding. It built the confidence of the power of using mobile for health and also development. Soon after, a number of programs followed that included:

- **Providing Comprehensive Holistic Care to Clients with TB, HIV/AIDS, and Cancer**, a program implemented with Kawempe Home Care (Hope Clinic Lukuli, Uganda) and funded by USAID between April 2010 and December 2010. The main focus of the program was to use text messages to increase utilization of health services (i.e. HIV/AIDS care, maternal care, and family planning) and communicate about health products available at Hope Clinic Lukuli. The evaluation results showed an increased adherence after SMS use: 87 per cent adherence above 95 per cent at project start and 93 per cent after 3 months. A testimonial from the partner highlights the success of the project: 'A greatly successful project as seen in the evaluation results, the clients adherence increased, their viral load reduced and their CD4 also went up.'
- **Using SMS to provide information on HIV/AIDS Prevention, Malaria, Family Planning, Medical Male Circumcision (MMC), Multiple Sexual Partnerships Health Initiatives for the Private Sector** (HIPS – Uganda), implemented from August 2009 (TTC, 2010). Under this Initiative, TTC has worked with four Ugandan companies: Kinyara Sugar in Masindi, Kakira Sugar Works in Jinja, Kasese Cobalt KCCL in Kasese, and Eskom Uganda. The program has seen a total of over 1,500 participants receiving about forty HIV/AIDS-related quizzes over a mobile phone, which has been coupled with VCT encouragement and company information sharing. The successes lies in having workers being able to timely and interactively participate in receiving and sharing health information via a mobile phone without leaving their workplaces. A research study is also under way to test the effectiveness of this program.

Many more programs have successfully followed the above that carry interesting results which we have continuously shared on our website (texttochange.com). These programs have attracted a large share of funding with the most recent where TTC will work with Connect4Change (C4C), a consortium funded by the Dutch Ministry of Foreign Affairs that brings together the expertise of five organizations in the field of development and ICT: AKVO, Cordaid, Edukans, ICCO, and IICD. C4C addresses the issues of poverty and exclusion in Africa and Latin America, in the areas of health, economic development, and education – seeking solutions based on the use of the internet and mobile phones. TTC has been identified as the partner of choice to complement these activities. Over the next five years from 2011, TTC will work with C4C and their local partners in Ghana, Malawi, Tanzania, Uganda, Zambia, Bolivia, Burkina Faso, Ethiopia, Kenya, Peru, and Mali.

TTC has, over the past four years, proven that **SMS and Voice**-based applications can be used successfully in various interactive mobile health education programs reaching thousands of people across the African continent. TTC has proved that the use of SMS to encourage behavior change is a highly effective communication channel for health education, encouraging testing and drug compliance and informing people of the choices available to them concerning their well-being. We are currently expanding from providing not only a platform for SMS and voice but also data collection.

Today, TTC is active in Uganda, Kenya, Tanzania, Namibia, Cameroon, and Sierra Leone and in the Democratic Republic of Congo (DRC) and is now expanding outside Africa to South America. We currently have strong partnerships with USAID, Airtel Bharti (formerly Zain), UNICEF, Family Health International (FHI), IICD, Infectious Disease Institute (IDI), Malaria Consortium, Health Child, Jpiegho, and the Dutch Ministry of Foreign Affairs, among others. TTC now employs a team of six employees in Uganda and six others in the Amsterdam office who carry a wealth of experience in program management and implementation.

Opportunities, Challenges, and lessons learned

The mobile landscape in Africa has since evolved over the past decade with 380 million mobile subscribers and one million added every week (Gartner Inc., 2011). This growth has been fueled in a large part by the liberalization effort, resulting in the formation of independent regulatory bodies and increased competition in the market. This has enhanced numerous grassroot efforts to empower the poor and marginalized by providing access to knowledge through technology, more so a platform for communication. SMS and voice is being used in innovative ways to share knowledge and improve learning in Africa.

Sixty per cent of people in Africa are currently under the age of twenty-four. This is a population that is knowledgeable about new technologies (growing to the use of smartphones) and demanding it. The end-users are booming with lots of enthusiasm to explore and learn any technologies at their disposal in schools and communities. They like to learn and are inquisitive (Hoefman, 2011). Bas says his idea is keeping it simple to encourage knowledge sharing. He has since also observed that mobile is still a more affordable technology compared other information-sharing tools for the masses seeing that service providers always have subsidized packages that accommodate various classes of people.

At the beginning of 2008, the 'mHealth' (mobile health) scene barely existed. TTC took advantage of this and piloted its SMS health campaigns in Uganda, on a large scale. Though the pilot was successful overall, 'everything that could have gone wrong, did go wrong...', including the fact that TTC had registered a short code with the number '666' that roused a negative impact among the clients. They saw this as a number of the devil and discouraged people from joining this campaign. This was the first major setback as we had to acquire a different figure for the short code. We used '777' instead. However, changing the short code number from 666 to 777 was not communicated well, which led to some participants pulling out because the activity was not clear to them. A lack of an introductory message about the service hindered the understanding of the program and affected participation. All the messages were sent in English, which created problems for non-English-speaking participants. The participants who selected the wrong answer to the multiple-choice questions were not always given the right answers. As the service provider, AIC, Mbarara branch, was not mentioned in the messages as the destination for the HCT services, and this led to some participants going elsewhere.

Above all, however, the results of the pilot established TTC as a major player in mHealth in Africa as well as paving the way for many others. TTC has along the way explored mobile growth opportunities to create brands such as the Mobile for Reproductive Health (M4RH) that has inbuilt innovative reproductive health packages. These packages have now become strong household names that have attracted opportunities for scale up to other countries. The opportunities of using mobile as a tool for health are currently numerous and endless. TTC has seen the rise of many mHealth competitors along the way but these have only made them think outside the box and explore new ideas – like presently data collection over a mobile phone and mobile marketing.

The rollout of mHealth has equipped us with various lessons that we share with enthusiasm:

- **Low literacy levels, especially in rural Africa.** SMS is often coupled with literacy – it requires the ability of the end-user to at least be able to read and write. Most times we have encountered mixed feelings from partners in this regard. However, TTC has encouraged that since an SMS is viral, an end-user can be assisted by sharing the information with another who is more literate.
- **Mobile operators are always seeking a win-win market situation.** How then should we package mHealth programs to make them interesting to the mobile operators? We also need to ask ourselves, can the people pay for health information? Mobile operators seek to make profits. At the moment, all TTC programs are funded by the responsible partner and that is why we can be able to sustain the cost of SMS. TTC has partnerships with most major mobile operators in East Africa from which we get subsidized tariffs. Our short codes run on all networks in Uganda, Kenya, and Tanzania. For example, Orange is providing us with technical support in countries where they have operations; however, the partnership does not demand exclusivity – we are open to work with other existing operators within the region.
- **Africa is characterized by too many mHealth pilots**, of which most have not materialized to ongoing, impact-generating programs. Many pilots in developing countries are currently donor funded and have created vast impact. The question is: *If they are successful, how do we plan to scale them up nationally or even all over Africa?* TTC has carried out numerous pilots and we are happy to note that a few have been identified for scale up to as far as other African countries. The secret lies in creating a program that can easily be scalable to other countries and communities. TTC has always worked with a model where the end-user is not paying for the services and the organization issuing the demand is responsible for part of the funding. TTC has established long-term funding agreements with Western agencies to secure a sustainable future for small programs that are being requested for by African organizations.
- **Low rural mobile penetration still remains a constant factor.** Much as we recognize and celebrate the growth of mobile presence, the reality is still a myth to rural populations in Africa. We found out that families in rural areas shared a mobile phone unit of which, more often than not,

ownership is bound to the male. This becomes a challenge in instances where information must be disseminated to the maler, reminding her about her antenatal care appointments to the clinic. Cultural norms such as these are still a strong and respectable factor in the African setting that cannot easily be reversed. Even when mobile unit presence would be improved, this would still be hampered by the scarcity of electricity availability in rural areas. TTC has found that in implementing some of the programs, we have to provide a solar charger together with phones so as to ensure smooth continuity of the program's activities.

- **Nonexistence of a central referral health content/facts database.** TTC on several instances has been challenged with finding a 'one stop shop' for suitable health content. Even so, designing content that can be shared with the limited 160 characters of an SMS is a tedious process. Even after a program has commenced, we find that it would take at least a few extra months before we actually begin because we have to go through a content collection and revision process. TTC has now resorted to create and store a databank of any relevant information that we come across at conferences, on the web, in books, and in magazines. After working with European research institutes and universities on health content to be sent out in Africa, all our post-pilot programs contain content that is developed by African organization, localized with regard to cultural, religious, and demographic differences.

Reflections and recommendations

Africa is currently a hotbed of mobile phone activity. The mobile phone is the new and exciting technique to reach out to people in Africa and that is why it cannot be flouted anymore. The continent has grown over the years to be mobile and this will only expand to include various uses. That was different when TTC started in 2007/2008, when only a few hundred people owned and maintained a mobile phone. Organizations enthusiastic to implement mHealth should ask themselves: *What problem is mobile going to solve for us? And what has already been done by other organizations?* Do not just use mobile because it is fashionable. We have learned that mHealth is not just about adding an mHealth component to an existing program or campaign; however, this needs to be integrated and planned from conception. One of the biggest challenges we have faced is the creation of content and the actual management of mHealth programs. The advice we always give to some of the organizations: do not think about the technology but let us know your challenges so that together we can decide if mobile will act as a solution. The challenges are: *How do you get people to work with it? And who is going to pay for it in the long run?*

The future of ICT/mobile phone deployment in health is encouraging and growing steadily; however, this cannot be substituted for a weak health economic system – a good quality and fully equipped health sector is vital. It should be understood that ICTs/mobile phones are just a tool or an enabler to economic development. We believe the biggest opportunities lie in the access to quality and timely health information and knowledge.

In our view, government should not be mandated to implement mHealth, but act as the overseer giving support and guidance as much as possible. They should also create an auspicious environment to deploy mHealth by putting policy frameworks and avail essential information and knowledge as often as they can. Approximately four years ago, TTC gave an eye-opening presentation about the potential of using mobile phones in health communication to senior management at the Ministry of Health in Uganda and from there on it was decided that mHealth was going to be used in their programs. We are afraid that this idea is a 'still born' birth culminating from long bureaucratic tendencies that run through ministries and governments.

Development of a strong regulatory framework involving a range of stakeholders with accent on end-user involvement will bring us far. For example, in Uganda a technical working group is in place with the aim to bring different stakeholders together to accelerate ICT implementations in Uganda. A national ICT policy is in place and a health sector ICT policy (eHealth) is already operational. The Uganda Ministry of Health is taking steps to coordinate ICT development and has allocated resources to support implementation of its ICT strategy. Nationwide deployment of an mHealth application program could only be successful with the inclusion of government having a dedicated budget. That said, mHealth applications have the potential to improve and strengthen the current health system if integrated into an existing 'well-functioning' structure.

Since 2008, TTC has seen widespread success, reaching hundreds of thousands of people via their mobile phones with health information which has undoubtedly contributed to an increase of knowledge and behavior change noticeable in the uptake of people going for health services (HIV counseling and testing, circumcision, and antenatal care) after receiving our messages. TTC will be gradually shifting from a nonprofit organization to a social enterprise. We will continue to expand our mobile services to serve communities around the globe with (health) information. TTC will still be recognized as one of the leading players in the field of mobile for development with a strong brand but in a more adventurous structure. To ensure sustainability, a combination of nonprofit work will be interwoven with profit-generating assignments, while prohibiting a conflict of interest. We are at a helm of this venture and the future of mHealth and mobile phones for developments lies within public–private partnerships. A challenge still underlies in moving from a donor-funded pilot phase to commercially viable products. *Who is the owner of mobile for development and who is going to pay?* Constructing a sustainable ecosystem is fundamental. Mobile technology is a strong and affordable technique that will foster tangible development. Nothing can stop an idea whose time has come.

References

Calder Strategies (2007), 'Mobile Campaign Primer', http://calderstrategies.com/wordpress/mobile-101/ [Accessed 15 February 2012].

Gartner Inc. (2011), 'Gartner Says Worldwide Mobile Payment Users to Reach 141 Million in 2011', Stamford: CT: http://www.gartner.com/it/page.jsp?id=1749114 [Accessed 15 February 2012].

Hahn, J. (2011), 'Can We Text Our Way to Behavior Change?', http://www.grameenfoundation.applab.org/blog/can-we-text-our-way-to-behavior-change.html [Accessed 15 February 2012].

Hoefman, B. (2011), 'Opportunities and Challenges for Use of Mobile Phones for Learning', https://edutechdebate.org/affordable-technology/opportunities-and-challenges-for-use-of-mobile-phones-for-learning/ [Accessed 15 February 2012].

ITU. (2009), 'Mobile Phone Subscribers Reach the Mark of 8.2 Mn (Uganda)', http://www.itu.int/ITU-D/ict/newslog/Mobile+Phone+Subscribers+Reach+The+Mark+Of+82Mn+Uganda.aspx [Accessed 15 February 2012].

ITU. (2010), *Mobile Health Solutions for Developing Countries*, Geneva: ITU.

Kasozi, J. and Basudde, E. (2008), 'Dutch Organisation to Fight AIDS with Mobile Phones', *The New Vision Uganda*.

McNamara, S. (2007), 2007 Africa – Telecoms, Internet and Mobile Statistics.

Nafula, J. (2008), 'Mobile Phones to Be Used in AIDS Fight', *The Daily Monitor (Uganda)*. Kampala.

Orth, B. (2011), Surfing the Gbps Wave, *CeBIT 2011*, Deutsche Telekom.

Royal Tropical Institute. (2010), 'The Impact of Text Message Quiz Programmes in Uganda', *mHealth in Low-Resource Settings*, http://www.mhealthinfo.org/impact-text-message-quiz-programmes-uganda [Accessed 15 February 2012].

TTC. (2010), 'Usaid, Hips and Text to Change to Launch HIV/AIDS Prevention and Health Promotion in the Workplace', http://www.texttochange.org/news/usaid-hips-and-text-change-launch-hivaids-prevention-and-health-promotion-workplace [Accessed 15 February 2012].

Uganda Bureau of Statistics (2006), *2006 Uganda Demographic and Health Survey*, Kampala: Gvt of Uganda.

11 Freedom HIV/AIDS

Mobile phone games for health communication and behavior change

Subhi Quraishi and Hilmi Quraishi, ZMQ Software Systems, India

Introduction

Freedom HIV/AIDS is a mobile games-based initiative (intervention) developed by ZMQ, a Technology for Development company in India. The initiative is designed to create information, awareness, and behavior change among the youths on issues related to sexual interaction, myths, and misconception surrounding HIV/AIDS, combating discrimination, and testing and treatment behaviors.

In 2004 and 2005, India was engulfed with an HIV/AIDS pandemic, with 5.13 million people living with HIV/AIDS then (UNAIDS, 2006). ZMQ launched 'Freedom HIV/AIDS' on December 1, 2005, the World AIDS Day, as a gift to Indian youths. ZMQ partnered with the state of Delhi, the Delhi State AIDS Control Society, and Reliance Infocomm – one of the largest mobile operators in India. Over the period, many more partners from all sectors joined the initiative to make it a success. Later, the initiative was scaled to different parts of Africa under the Africa Reach program of ZMQ. The success of the initiative led the company to start many more new mobile games initiatives to address critical health challenges in the developing world.

One of the strategies adopted was to create four games to catch different mindsets of people, games targeting youths, rural communities, and out-of-school children, using popular and accessible games, clear and well-designed messages, easy to maneuver user interfaces, and clear instructions.

On the first day of the campaign, mobile games on HIV/AIDS were made available to 29 million subscribers of Reliance. Later, more telecom operators were added. In a span of three years, the games reached 42 million subscribers with 10.3 million game sessions downloaded. This initiative was among the first and the largest mobile phone game program in the world to create behavior change.

In this chapter, we first outline the development of the games; second, link them to various impacts such as learning and behavior change; third, discuss some ways we measured the impact of the games, and fourth, discuss various challenges of the projects – both internal and external.

Objectives

The objective of the program was to reach out to the youths to increase their knowledge about HIV and AIDS, with the broader goal of encouraging behavior changes, including:

- Promoting abstinence from sexual activity until marriage to increase the age of sexual debut.
- Promoting the importance of being faithful to reduce the number of partners.
- Increasing the correct and consistent use of Condoms.
- Improving knowledge of HIV and other STI transmissions.
- Reducing myths and misconceptions.
- Reducing the level of stigma and discrimination associated with people living with HIV/AIDS.
- Increasing the demand for information and services related to HIV and AIDS.

Why mobile?

Mobile is a device for almost everyone. It is an ideal tool for interventions targeting individuals, especially the youth. The reach of mobile phones in developing countries is more than any other technology or infrastructure. There has been a tremendous growth in the number of low-resource handsets in the world, and the growing penetration of telecom networks especially in the developing world. People who never had access to technologies such as fixed landline phones, computer, or the internet, now have mobile phones in their hands for communication and data transfer. According to the prime UN telecommunications agency, International Telecommunication Union, the number of mobile phone subscriptions worldwide has reached 4.6 billion and is expected to increase to five billion. India alone has over 750 million mobile phone subscribers (ITU, 2010). This explosion of mobile phone usage especially in developing countries has the potential to service delivery on a massive scale.

We believe that exploiting the ubiquity of mobile phones and taking information through mobile phones to communities at a massive level can improve their lives. This was done by turning critical information into an approachable language using mobile phone games and integrating them in the public health management system to connect with communities on issues related to HIV/AIDS and other communicable diseases.

Theory of change: mobile games as an effective tool for learning and behavior change

From card games to puppetry to video games, people have been playing games for centuries. A game is a challenge posed for users, which provides engagement to players with some target/objective to be achieved, based on some set of rules and frameworks. A player needs to perform different tasks which he/she would be unable to perform in the real world. Thus, the virtual activity of the game enables the player to engage in a risk-based activity of the real world in a virtual risk-free environment. This risk-free environment gives an opportunity to the player to try various risk options of the real world and see the consequence of each of them without any physical harm. This virtual environment also helps the user to learn new things, de-learn the previously learned things, and apply new things based on the cognitive learning, which leads to behavior change in the virtual world, thus retaining the changed behavior in the real world.

Our theory of change has been the use of mobile phone games to create awareness on HIV and AIDS, finally leading to behavior change. It has been proven that games can serve as an ideal platform to provide real-world environments and its risks on a compact (in terms of both resources and timeline), risk-free platform. The game enhances knowledge and learning in an engaging and entertainment mode, and this provides a basis for promoting behavior change. The complete model of learning for behavior change in the world of digital games is based on social cognitive theory (Baranowski, Buday, Thomson, and Baranowski, 2007).

The theory proposes that behavior change is a function of enhanced skills and confidence in doing the new behavior. Games engage users and add elements of enjoyment and excitement, thereby enhancing behavior change through enhanced motivation. The use of mobile phone games for health-related behavior change is still in the early stage of development, but incorporating theory-based change procedures provides reason to believe that they can be effective.

Models of behavior change communication in Freedom HIV/AIDS games

Freedom HIV/AIDS has taken inspirations from various behavior change theories such as social cognitive theory, AIDS risk reduction model, health belief model, and the stages of change. The approach adopted by ZMQ has been more of a blended approach, by taking some components from these theories and embedding them in the games. Drawing on an array of genres, content types, and learning activities outlined by Prensky (Prensky, 2001), our research team explored various game formats such as participatory games, board games, and online games to understand and adopt various strategies in designing the games. Some of the genres which were taken as inspiration were role-play games, decision-making games, detective games, single shooter game, popular sports-based games, virtual game shows, and action mini-games.

ZMQ has also been studying the behavioral patterns of its previous games and at the same time regularly launching more and new genres of games to have a better understanding of behavioral patterns. One thing that has been observed common among all these games has been the interaction with various real-world scenarios in a risk-free gaming environment. This has been named as '*Real-World Risk Reduction Method using Game Mechanics*' – a ZMQ model.

Other key considerations

One of the key considerations to develop the gaming campaign was to have games available on low-end devices. It was important to develop games for black and white devices which had a very small cache memory, as 65 per cent of Reliance subscribers were based in semi-urban and rural areas with low-end devices. The challenge was to keep the game size to 32 kilobytes for black and white and 64 kilobytes for colored devices. Another key consideration was to have simple messages and user-friendly instructions. Lots of icon-based messages were also used to convey messages to less literate communities. One of the other main reasons to use cricket and quizes was the same. People in India know how to play cricket, and trivia game shows (based on 'Who wants to be a Millionaire') have been popular TV shows/games in India for years. The game design in terms of maneuverability was kept simple, user-friendly, and easy. Also the instructional designing of the game was done in a scientific method. One of the other main considerations in designing the game was to keep intact cultural values. In the Indian context, giving HIV/AIDS information and talking about sex are considered taboo, so the messages were designed keeping the cultural sensitivities in mind.

The games

Safety cricket – a mass appeal game

One of the games planned to be used for Freedom HIV/AIDS was decided to be a sports-based genre. Cricket is the most popular sport in India. It is like a religion in this part of the world. The game is played and watched by almost everyone – the rich and poor, young and old, men and women. Safety Cricket has been a very popular and mass appeal game based on cricket.

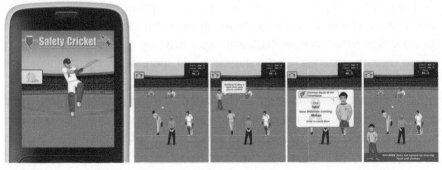

Figure 11.1 Screenshot of Safety Cricket
Source: Freedom HIV/AIDS and ZMQ

As the majority of the people know the rules of the game, users playing a mobile game do not need any specific instructions to understand the game play. But then there was another reason, more of a scientific one than anything else, of choosing cricket as our prime game for the initiative. This is primarily the format of the game, which involves different game mechanisms; bowling – in different styles, batting – with different strokes, scoring different types of runs, getting out in different styles, fielding, and wicket keeping. It is also a turn-based game, where two teams play their innings in turns and eleven players of each team play one by one to make one innings. The playing style of one batsman can really influence the behavior of other batsmen, thus inducing a certain sense of precaution before taking a risk, which matches with the social learning theory of behavior change (Bandura, 1977).

The first component of learning in the game is an informational component, which gives knowledge to the players and increases awareness on HIV and related risk. The messages clearly demonstrated how a risky shot played by a batsman can bowl him out from the game and similarly in a real-life scenario too. The messages were simple but clear to impart learning, create awareness, and increase knowledge.

Another component in the game related to the social theory is to develop self-control and risk-reduction skills. The cricket game helped the player to know what their risks are and how they can change them. In the cricket game, risk balls in the game need to be tackled very carefully. The player needs to take adequate precaution while playing the ball and try to reduce risk in selecting shots and develop self-control. The player should also learn how to leave a ball which might look like a loose ball but actually is misleading and can be fatal. Similar situations are enacted in the real-life scenario, especially related to risky sex behaviors.

The third component in the game is to increase an individual's self-efficacy in implementing these behaviors. Self-efficacy helps in developing an individual's character by imbibing learning from observing things and experiencing various different situations. This component helped users to enhance their skills like how to use condoms correctly, how to negotiate safer sex, and how to say no to unpleasant situations or unwilling circumstances. The cricket game play did it in the same manner. The game was designed as a single player game, but was used in two ways. In the first mode, the game was played by single users in an individual game play mode, and in the second mode, it was played as a single-player shared game in community settings in a group of four to ten people. The first mode was predominantly used by individuals downloading and playing the game. Here, a player would role-play as different batsmen and learn from the previous batsman's mistakes and improve in consecutive batting turns. Thus, the user learns by observing multiple batting styles and different risk-plays, thus gradually correcting in consecutive batting turns. The batsman trying to attempt a risky and fast (deadly) ball is likely to get out.

The community shared game-play mode was primarily used for training in the classrooms and group meetings. Here, the game was played in group settings of four to ten players who played a single game by turns and sharing the same device. The player batting first is observed by the next batter in the turn. The consecutive batsman observes the playing styles and risks in the game, and tries to improve on mistakes by imitating a safer-play. On every fall of wicket, the outgoing player will share his mode of getting out with his peers and discuss the messages he received during the game-play. The discussion helped the players to model perfect game-play style to win the game. The group mode also helped in improving an individual's performances.

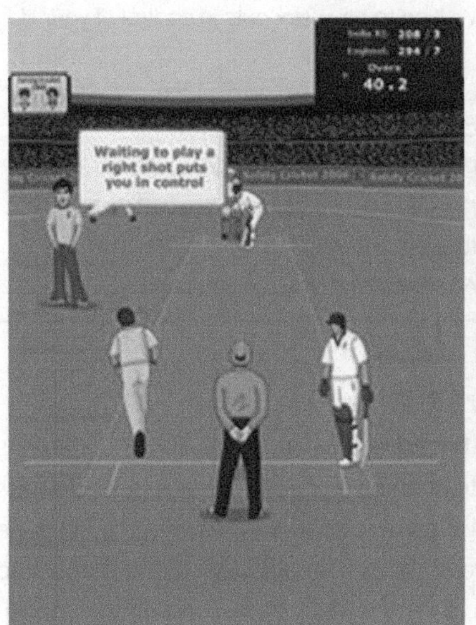

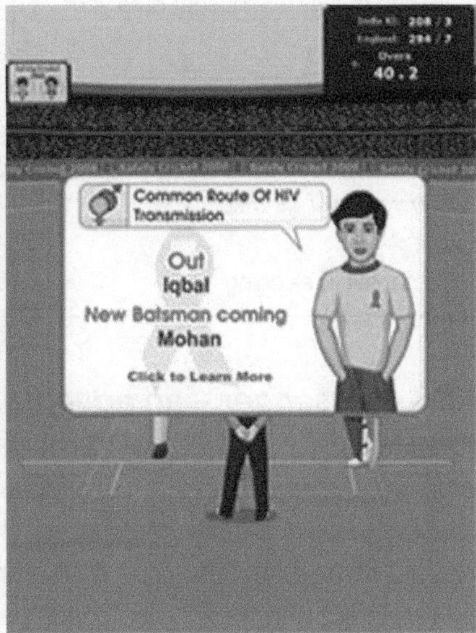

Figure 11.2 Screenshot of Safety Cricket messages
Source: Freedom HIV/AIDS and ZMQ

Cricket was just a tool to pull the crowd to play the game but the messages played a crucial role in associating different cricketing instances with a real-life risks and situations related to HIV and AIDS. For instance, a message like '*No Helmet No Cricket; No Condom No Sex*' became popular slogan and jingle.

Below is the list of cricketing messages alongside the subsequent life-based (HIV/AIDS) messages used in the game.

Table 11.1 Messages used in the game

Cricketing Messages	HIV/AIDS Messages
Flirting with outgoing deliveries could get you out	Saying Yes to abstinence is saying Yes to oneself
Protect yourself by wearing a guard and a helmet	Use condoms for safe sex
Play with caution	Be faithful to one partner – prevent HIV/AIDS
Play carefully. Do not step out of crease	Abstinence protects you from HIV and STDs
Be careful, do not run your partner out	Love means faithful to one partner
Take your time. Do not rush	Irresponsible behavior can lead to HIV/AIDS
Saying No to risk means saying Yes to your team	Be faithful and make a happy family
Select a right delivery to avoid risks	Avoid unsafe and casual sex
Waiting to play a right shot puts you in control	Waiting to have sex puts in control of your life
Do not hurry, build a partnership	Enjoy a relationship without the complications of sex
Take your own time to score run	Do not fall to peer pressure
Play your innings well	Do not hurry for sex, abstinence is the best to avoid HIV/AIDS
Do not fall to sledging	Avoid unwanted sexual attention

AIDS Messenger – an adventure game

AIDS Messenger game is an adventure-based multilevel game. From a gamer's perspective, this is simple to play, easy to maneuver, highly engaging, and offers instant rewards. Moreover, the speed of the game-play increased with the increase in levels, which made the game even more exciting. The objective of the game is to deliver correct objects such as condoms, safe sex instructions, red ribbon, health tips, access to blood tests (HIV testing), counseling tips, and tips to reduce stigma to virtual communities in the game, based on their specific needs and risk assessments.

The behavior change induced in the game has taken inspiration from the AIDS Risk Reduction Model (ARRM) developed by Catania, Kegeles and Coates (1990). In the AIDS Messenger game, the player moves from one level to the next level in the game, as a result of delivery of correct information and safety objects demanded by the virtual communities and villagers. The gamers must pass through three stages – identifying demands of villagers (behavior labeling), selection of right objects for delivery (commitment to change), and making the right delivery at the right time (action).

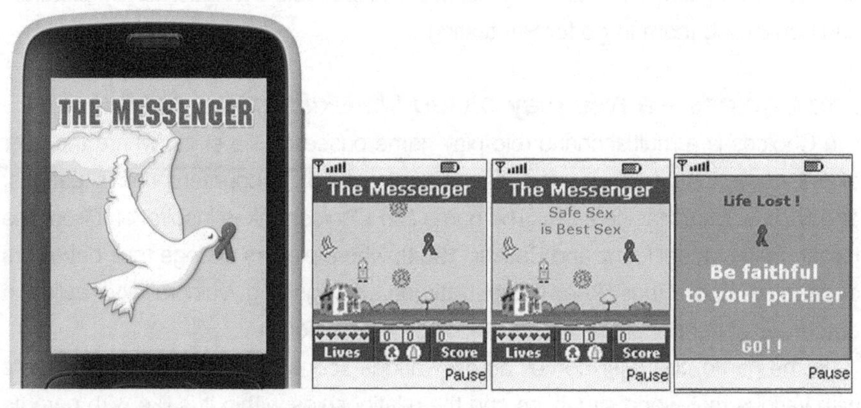

Figure 11.3 Screenshot of The Messenger
Source: Freedom HIV/AIDS and ZMQ

In the game, the user is represented in the form of a dove – a symbol of peace or a messenger of HIV/AIDS awareness. In the gaming mode, the user goes around various virtual communities and identifies risk behaviors in every community. The people in various such communities are engaged in different types of risk behaviors such as IDUs engaged in use of drugs and alcohol, youths engaged in unsafe sexual activities, truck drivers having unsafe sex, female sex workers having sex with multiple partners, migrant workers engaged in unsafe sexual practices and being unfaithful to their wives, and men having sex with men engaged in unsafe sex and having multiple partners. These are all labeled as high risk members as they are involved in high risk activities, which can transmit HIV and AIDS. This is the stage where an individual's behavior in the community is recognized and is labeled as high risk behavior. Thus in the game, the risk assessment process immediately informs the communities about high risks in their life and the gamer tags these communities.

In the next level of the game, these tagged community members are immediately advised to check their activities, based on risk assessment in the first level of the game. This is simply done by providing them timely advisory services with powerful messages to influence and then change their actions and behavior by counseling them, providing health tips, increasing their knowledge related to HIV/AIDS and STIs, and busting the myths on the use of condoms. Thus in this stage, players are counseled and are asked to make a commitment to reduce high-risk sexual activities and to increase low risk activities.

Finally, in the last level of the game, if community members in the game do not change their risk styles, they are approached with a focused virtual action to change their behaviors. The idea is to take action, which is provided in the game through the use of virtual avatars with messages, the users are provided with condoms, accelerated counseling services, disposable syringes, family pictures, and convincing them to go for HIV testing.

Life Choices – a role play based life-skills game for girls

Life Choices is a multiscenario role-play game based on life skills, where the user examines various feelings, negotiates relationships, encounters risk situations, and finds ways to tackle them. The game *Life Choices* takes inspirations from the Health Belief Model (Janz and Becker, 1984), where players change their behaviors depending upon their knowledge, attitude, recognizing vulnerability, belief in outcomes of right choices, and by taking prompt action.

In the game, the user comes across various scenarios where he/she interacts with various real-world situations and the relationships within it is like with parents at home, relatives and cousins, peers in school, boyfriends/girlfriends, friends at a party, and people in public places such as transport (bus and metro) and mall

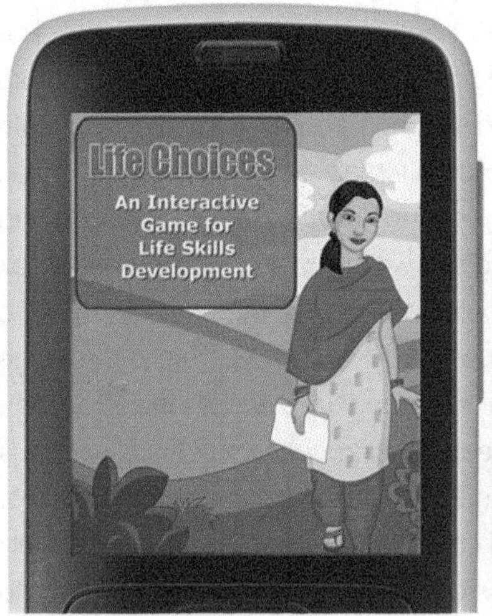
Life Choices
An Interactive Game for Life Skills Development

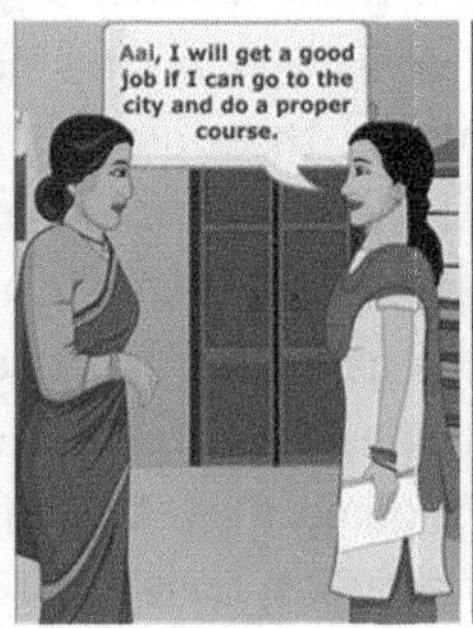
Aai, I will get a good job if I can go to the city and do a proper course.

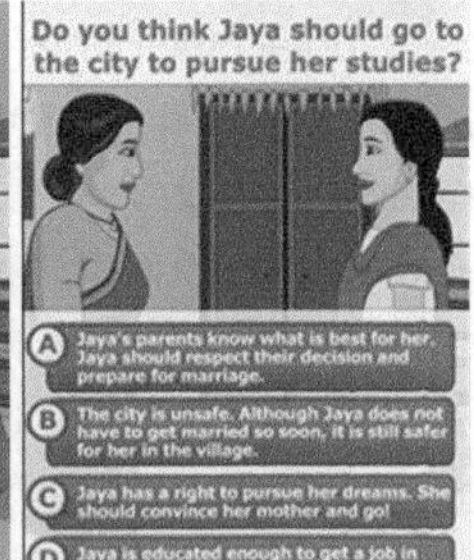
Do you think Jaya should go to the city to pursue her studies?
A Jaya's parents know what is best for her. Jaya should respect their decision and prepare for marriage.
B The city is unsafe. Although Jaya does not have to get married so soon, it is still safer for her in the village.
C Jaya has a right to pursue her dreams. She should convince her mother and go!
D Jaya is educated enough to get a job in the village.

Figure 11.4 Screenshot of Life Choices
Source: Freedom HIV/AIDS and ZMQ

(carnival and shops). Each situation presents a dilemma and alternative course of action that a user has to choose from. On selecting an option, the user examines the possible consequences of each situation. In each situation, the user also has to examine various feelings and negotiate various relationships. The main character in the game is a girl, whose objective in life is to achieve her professional goals. In order to achieve this, she encounters different real-life challenging situations and examines her feelings, negotiates relationships with peers and friends, communicates with her parents and teachers, explores various feelings of attraction, establishes relationships with partners, and often restrains her feelings. For instance, in one of the situations, the mother of the girl persuades her to get married early. The situation depicts emotional pressure from the mother and the rest of the family. The girl examines all the consequences of getting married early and has choices to select for the next step. The objective of the scenario is to negotiate family pressure and find a correct step to move to the next situation. In this scenario, the correct step is to pursue her education further and acquire professional skills to lead a healthier, happier life.

The game provides different options and the user selects one of the options and sees its consequence. Any option chosen whose consequence is negative and arouse a warning will lead to change in attitude and ultimately change in related behavior.

Great Escape – a role play based detective game

Great Escape is a role-play based detective game and takes some inspiration from two models of behavior change; partly from the stages of change model (Prochaska, DiClimente and Norcross, 1992) and partly from the social learning theory.

In the game, the user is a detective who is trapped in different risk situations and needs to fix solutions in each situation and find an ultimate escape route to win the game. In this process, the detective (user) passes through various risk situations – one after another to ultimately make a successful escape. The stages of change model is embedded at the micro-level of the game play that is within each game level (risk scenario) and the components of social learning theory are woven at the macro-level (learning shared across different risk scenarios).

Each situation in the game is a micro-level scenario where the detective (user) first has to identify the scenario and the risk associated with it. He then has to find relevant tools to solve the problem in that situation. For instance – if the user is trapped in a network of intravenous drug users (IDUs), he first needs to identify the risk situation (pre-contemplation) and then he needs to identify danger sign (contemplation), that is sharing of syringes or use of re-use of syringes in this scenario. Finally, the user has to provide the right tools (action), for example searching disposable syringes and relevant counseling tips.

At the macro-level, moving from one situation to another, the user collects tools to identify each scenario, its problems, and solutions. For instance, in the IDU scenario, the user finds condoms or counseling booklets for the truckers which he does not use in the present scenario but carries it forward to be used in other appropriate risk scenarios. Thus the user is using his previous learning and applying it in the subsequent risk situations.

As the core mechanics of the game is of a detective game genre, the user also has to search, collect, and use escape tools such as keys, maps, mobile phones, a passport, credit card, password, and other items that help him in his ultimate escape. These escape tools are collected by answering questions correctly (HIV/AIDS quiz), presented in a quizzing format (as a trivia game) with four options based on the style of popular game show 'Who wants to be a Millionaire'.

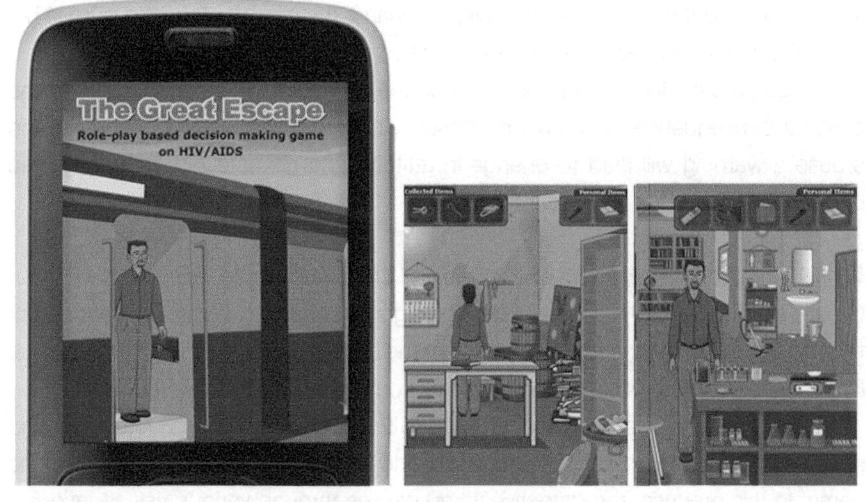
The Great Escape
Role-play based decision making game on HIV/AIDS

Figure 11.5 Screenshot of The Great Escape
Source: Freedom HIV/AIDS and ZMQ

Evaluation

The games designed had different outcomes in general. The learning outcomes from the games designed have been immense. Safety Cricket game resulted in change is various risks behaviors based on learning from observation and dealing with the consequences. Some of the key outcomes were increased use of condoms (safer sex methods), increased debut age for having sex (abstinence), and reduction in number of partners (being faithful). The outcome of AIDS messenger game was based on the actions generated by identifying risk behavior and then delivering the right message. The game resulted in adopting safer sex practices, especially the use of condoms by busting the general perception that the use of condom reduces the sexual enjoyment. There was also increasing interest to visit counseling and HIV testing centers.

Life Choices was popular with adolescent girls. It increased the negotiating and decision-making skills of the adolescent girls, and helped them take their own decisions without any peer pressure. The negative consequences in the game aroused a warning, leading to change in attitude and ultimately change in behaviors related to life and health. In the game The Great Escape, the user identifies a risk situation, recognizes the need to change the situation, tries to acquire the tools to change, and maintains the same behavior if similar situation occurs. The overall outcome of the games increased safer sex practices and enhanced decision-making capabilities.

Assessing learning

Study 1

The method adopted to see the impact of mobile games was by conducting live workshops and doing sample surveys. Four villages in the outskirts of Allahabad, Saharanpur, Patna, and Sholapur were selected. In every region, 200 to 300 children from local schools, settlements, and out-of-school children were invited for a two-day workshop. Initially, children were asked to answer questions related to HIV/AIDS. Their answers were assessed. Later children were given instructions to play mobile games on HIV/AIDS. Each group was divided into four sub-groups where they were made to play each game three times. Depending upon the game,

Table 11.2 Co-efficient of learning summary results

Games	Pre-Test	Post-Test			Co-efficient of Learning after Three Game Sessions
		First Attempt	Second Attempt	Third Attempt	
Safety Cricket	.40	.48	.57	.68	.28
Great Escape	.33	.39	.46	.55	.22
Life Choices	.28	.37	.38	.49	.21
AIDS Messenger	.23	.24	.31	.38	.08
Average learning in all the games	.31	.37	.43	.51	.13

every child spent four to eight minutes per game. The initial learning was captured through pre-test. After every game-play, the children were given a post-test. The post-test comprises of five questions. Thus every game was played thrice and three post-tests were captured. The results demonstrated an increase in learning on a scale of one, after each game play, which is referred as co-efficient of learning in our survey. The survey demonstrated that there was an evident increase in learning from a pre-test score of 0.31 to 0.56 after the third game-play.

Study 2

The launch of the games was primarily an open-ended approach. In the span of fifteen months, the games reached to over 42 million subscribers with a real-time download of 10.3 million game sessions. A game session is defined as when the person has downloaded the game, played it, and submitted the score back on the server. There was a need to evaluate the game impact in a targeted sample region. For this, we used Safety Cricket, as it was a very special game which attracted a lot of people due to its popularity. In this game, a specialized social engine was built with pre-test and post-test models. This engine was used in a district for four weeks, where 27,900 users registered through a mass media campaign and over 76,000 game sessions of Safety Cricket were downloaded and played. The game starts with a pre-test form on HIV/AIDS with five questions on HIV/AIDS related to basics, transmission, and prevention with focus on safer sex practices, peer pressure, and sharing of syringes. After attempting the pre-test, the user plays the game. Every event in the game like scoring runs, getting out, or leaving a ball had its own category of messaging. Thus the arithmetical calculation of number of runs scored, wickets lost, balls played, and balls missed reflects types and number of messages delivered. After playing the game five times, a post-test form was generated with a

Table 11.3 Co-efficient of learning for Safety Cricket

Category of Messages Delivered	Pre-test Results	Delivery of Messages based on Category	Post-test Results
Basics on HIV/AIDS	0.57	18%	0.88
Transmission	0.39	31%	0.66
Prevention	0.43	23%	0.78
Testing	0.21	15%	0.43
Stigma	0.15	13%	0.44
Average Score	0.35	----	0.64

new set of questions. On completion, all the data related to pre-test, game sessions (five sessions), and post-test was submitted. This data was then analyzed.

Out of the 27,900 users registered in the survey, only 8,213 users played the games completely – submitting pre-test, playing it five times, and submitting the post-test. The average co-efficient of learning increased from 0.35 to 0.64. The results in Table 11.3 are based on the users playing it five times and then submitting the post-test.

Qualitative analysis was done to assess behavior change. Random surveys and interviews were conducted in the communities and audiences where the games were played. The success of the program was measured in terms of the following indicators.

- Increase in safer sex practices (condom usage, abstinence, faithfulness, and value of a single partner).
- Increase in ability and skills to fight peer pressure.
- Increase in demand for disposable syringes at healthcare facilities.
- General reduction in myths and misconceptions in the youths on issues related to HIV/AIDS.
- Reduction in stigma and discrimination against people living with HIV/AIDS.

Piloting and scale up

The mass media campaign started with the launch of mobile games on December 1, 2005 – the World AIDS Day and was inaugurated by Sheila Dikshit, the chief minister of Delhi. The games were made available to 27 million mobile subscribers of Reliance Infocomm, a leading mobile operator. At that time, 65 per cent subscribers of Reliance were based in rural India. In a span of three years, the games were available on other mobile operators and reached almost 42 million mobile phones with a real-time download of 10.3 million game sessions played. Almost 63 per cent of the games were played in smaller towns and cities. Analysis of these downloads in smaller towns and cities has shown that the prime reason of greater download was due to them being media-dark regions, where people did not have access to other mediums such as newspapers and TV.

Many parallel campaigns were also done using school learning games on HIV/AIDS in local languages, including Hindi, Marathi, Telugu, Kannada, Tamil, and Bengali. These campaigns became part of knowledge centers of the government of India (education department) with an additional 1.2 million beneficiaries. The project got extensive coverage in the media. Reliance also promoted the games by not only providing them free but also sending SMS messages to millions of customers on a weekly basis. The games were made available on the top category of Reliance R-World. This also enabled the successful dissemination of the games at a much larger scale. A lot of poster campaigns were done in schools, colleges, and also at mobile recharge centers. NGO workers were involved to promote the games while doing their own campaigns. The pre-test of the four games showed tremendous results. In span of fifteen months, over 10.3 million game sessions were played.

Freedom HIV/AIDS was replicated in East Africa. In December 2006, a new series of games on HIV/AIDS was launched in Kenya, Tanzania, and Uganda in local languages – Kiswahili and Shen – under ZMQ's Africa Reach Program. In two years' time, the games reached to over 6 million mobile handsets with a real-time download of 1.2 million game sessions played.

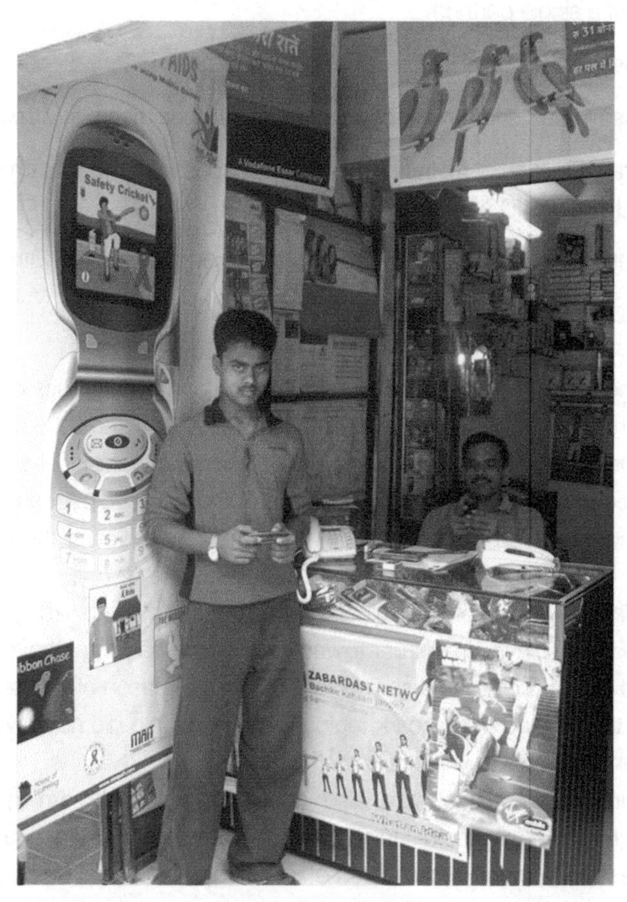

Figure 11.6 Poster campaign of freedom HIV/AIDS at mobile recharge kiosks in a semiurban location

Conclusion

Although India still has the largest number of people living with HIV in south and south-east Asia, the rate of new HIV infections has nevertheless fallen by 56 per cent (UNAIDS, 2011). ZMQ's games are not entirely responsible for this turnaround, but at scale, we are confident that our messaging was a positive contribution to the turning of the tides. More gaming exercises were done by ZMQ for other communicable diseases such as tuberculosis and malaria and other lifestyle diseases such as diabetes, chronic problems, and cancer. Overall, gaming is a successful approach to create effective learning outcomes and bring about behavior change, especially in the field of health.

Acknowledgments

We would like to thank Dr Ilmana Fasih for providing her valuable feedback on this paper. Dr Ilmana was also technical lead in developing HIV/AIDS content for the Freedom HIV/AIDS games. Also, we take this opportunity to thank Mr Jasdev Singh for creating the graphics and charts based on the pre-test and post-test reports. A special thanks to Ms Bupinder Singh, Secretary Health and Head Delhi State AIDS Control Society in 2005, state of Delhi and NCR, for the validation of content and helping in conducting pre-tests in the state.

References

Bandura, A. (1977), *Social Learning Theory*, Englewood Cliffs, NJ: Prentice Hall.

Baranowski, T., Buday, R., Thomson, D. and Baranowski, J. (2007), 'Playing for Real: Video Games and Stories for Health-Related Behavior Change', *American Journal of Preventive Medicine* 34(1): 74–82.

Catania, J., Kegeles, S. and Coates, T. (1990), 'Towards an Understanding of Risk Behavior: An AIDS Risk Reduction Model (ARRM)', *Health Education Quarterly* 17(1): 53–72.

ITU (2010), Free Statistics.

Janz, N. and Becker, M. (1984), 'The Health Belief Model: A Decade Later', *Health Education Quarterly* 11(1): 1–47.

Prensky, M. (2001), *Digital Game-Based Learning*, Columbus, OH: McGraw-Hill.

Prochaska, J., DiClimente, C. and Norcross, J. (1992), 'In Search of How People Change: Applications to Addictive Behaviors', *American Psychologist* 47(9): 1102–14.

UNAIDS (2006), 2006 Report on the Global AIDS Epidemic: A UNAIDS 10th Anniversary Special Edition.

UNAIDS (2011), *UNAIDS World AIDS Day Report 2011*, Geneva: UNAIDS.

12 Adhere.IO

José Gomez-Marquez, Massachusetts Institute of Technology

Introduction

Behavioral diagnostics can be a powerful force in persuasive behavior change and health. Our team at the MIT has developed and tested this new class of diagnostics aimed at improving medication adherence by remote for verification and persuasive incentives. Our platform called Adhere.IO began as a small student project called New Dots, later renamed XoutTB to reflect an application to improve tuberculosis medication adherence. Our journey into the use of mobile technology for behavior change began as a way of improving drug adherence to complex drug regimens, such as HIV and tuberculosis. We began by combining the latest findings from psychological and economic research and innovations in chemical and micro scale engineering to result in a combination diagnostic that uses lateral flow technology – the same biomedical technology that run pregnancy tests diagnostics – aided by mobile telephony.

Enabling patients to complete their treatment not only improves patient health directly, but also helps prevent the spread of drug-resistant strains of tubercular systems that are becoming more prevalent (Haynes, McDonald, Garg, and Montague, 2002).

Adhere.IO was invented at the MIT to introduce a new class of medical devices called behavioral diagnostics. Behavioral diagnostics combine emerging trends in applied behavioral economics and diagnostic design at the microscale wrapped in a telemedical application. Our application of behavioral diagnostics is a home-based test aimed at improving poor adherence of complex drug regimens such as HIV and tuberculosis, in low- and middle-income countries as well as high income countries. Our journey in developing behavioral diagnostics started with a challenge to improve TB medication adherence. We learned and are learning many lessons along the way.

The challenge

Tuberculosis (TB) remains a major public health concern more than sixty years after the first effective TB antibiotics were developed. According to the World

Health Organization (WHO), one-third of the global population is infected with tuberculosis bacillus, and 10 per cent will develop active tuberculosis. In 2010, there were roughly 8.8 million new cases of active TB and nearly 1.7 million TB deaths (WHO, 2011).

The conventional response: Treatment and adherence

TB treatment consists of a six- to nine-month course of antibiotics, usually a combination of isoniazid and rifampacin, taken orally (Centers for Disease Control and Prevention, 2009). Patients may often start treatment earnestly given that they may already be suffering from symptoms of the disease. As the antibiotics begin to do their job, the TB symptoms may begin to subside and the only remaining discomfort are the side effects of the medication itself. A qualitative visual representation of the problem is shown in Figure 12.1.

The system currently recommended by the WHO for tackling the problem of non-adherence is Directly Observed Therapy Short-Course (DOTS), which involves onsite, in-person monitoring of adherence with prescription drugs. Formal DOTS programs are often compromised and their performance is less than ideal. This is exacerbated by absenteeism and low attendance among community healthcare workers (Banerjee and Duflo, 2006; Chaudhury, Hammer, Kremer, Muralidharan, and Rogers, 2006). Furthermore, DOTS is a punitive measure that often results in a patient reprimand rather than peer support.

Community-based DOTS (CB-DOTS), using treatment partners as 'social capital' to ensure adherence, are protocols in which trained community members or peers observe the ingestion of each dose of medication (Ware, Idoko, Kaaya,

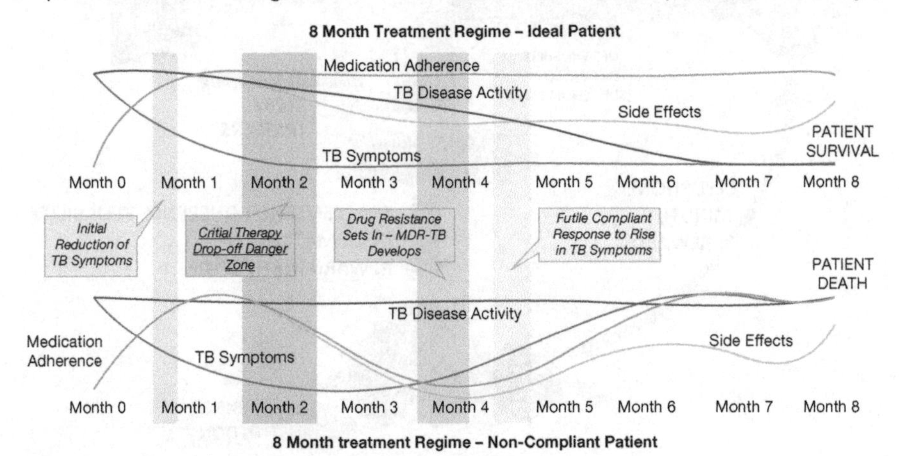

Figure 12.1 Visual representation of TB adherence

Biraro, Wyatt, Agbaji, Chalamilla, and Bangsberg, 2009); they have brought down the costs of DOTS but community programs vary considerably in their quality.

The WHO estimates that nearly 20 per cent of the world's population lives in areas still yet not covered by DOTS or similar programs (WHO, 2010). While most of these people will never develop cases of active TB, there exists a small portion who are at high risk for developing active TB because of latent TB infections or weakened immune systems. A cheap and effective monitoring technology that does not rely on health or community workers to see the patient every day has the potential to provide an effective yet inexpensive method for ensuring adherence in these vulnerable populations that do not have access to DOTS-like programs (Moulding, 2007). DOTS is estimated to cost US $120 per patient (Wandwalo, Robberstad and Morkve, 2005), Adhere.IO can cost as low as US $40–US $70 per patient.

Adhere.IO's approach to increasing adherence

Adhere.IO creates an interactive feedback loop using reminders, monitoring, and incentives, as shown in Figure 12.2.

At the heart of the system is a colorimetric diagnostic that reveals an alphanumeric secret code when exposed to the metabolites of a drug. In order to produce such metabolites, the drug has to be ingested and a sample, such as urine, placed on the test. Within minutes, the code is revealed as the chemicals from the test

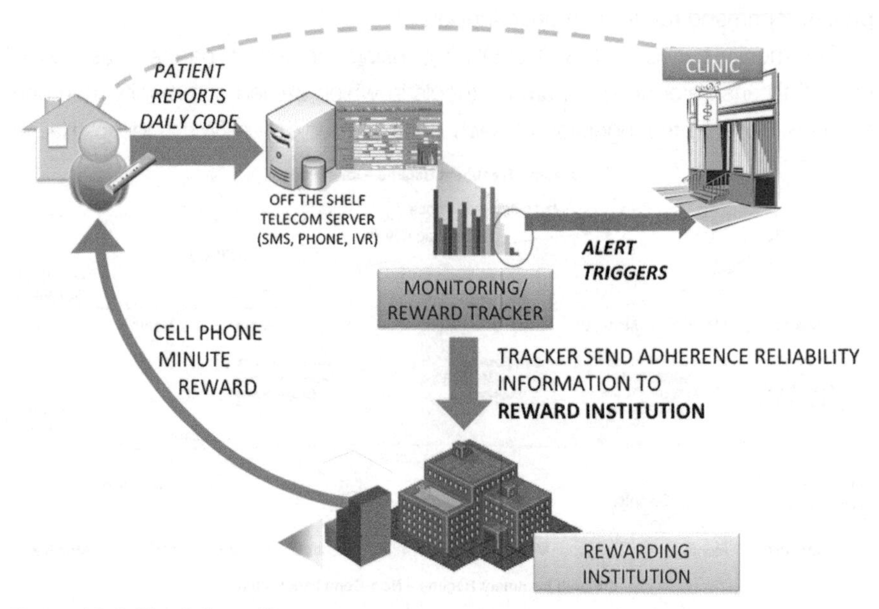

Figure 12.2 The Adhere.IO system

react with the metabolites. The test only reacts with the medication's metabolites, and only those metabolites, voiding the possibility of revealing the code without taking the medication. The patient will then send that code via SMS to a number linked to a database that matches the code to the expected answer. The patient receives a reward based on the correct codes that they send in (Gomez-Marquez and Hanumara, 2010).

Adhere.IO uses established lateral flow technology with a twist interactive diagnostics. Chromatography paper is formed into paper fluidic channels and embedded in chemicals that result in a colorimetric reaction not unlike a variant of the standard pH dipstick test. The technology is affordable, designed to be locally manufacturable, and because it is based on paper which is highly ubiquitous, easy to scale and distribute. It is also instrument free (as in the previous paragraph). In order to detect whether a drug is there, thus allowing the patient to reveal compliance at a distance, we need to detect one of the following, the metabolite of the drug, the drug itself, or potentially a tracer embedded on the drug, or an indirect ingredient already found in the drug. As a launching pad we chose to detect a metabolite commonly found in isoniazid which is isonicotinic acid which is excreted in urine. The reaction is commonly described as the Potts-Cozart reaction and is based off of many available commercial tests. We modified the published test into a paper diagnostic.

In practice, patients are given sets of test strips that they use every day to prove that they have taken their medication. Unlike DOTS where a healthcare worker intervenes to monitor, the patient sends his or her proof code via an SMS to a central processing database that tracks the patient's compliance rates. For each week that the patient succeeds in taking his or her medication, they receive a reward in the form of cellphone minutes (immediately transferred electronically to their cellphones). These short-term incentives aim to keep patients engaged in their long-term treatment. What this provides is a private benefit to the patient (an incentive such as cellphone minutes) as well a public benefit to both the patient (increased chance of survival) and society (decreased infection rates). What economists have long known is that people are more responsive to short-term private benefits faster than they do to public benefits. Economists call this hyperbolic discounting (Ainslie and Monterosso, 2002).

The evolution of our approach

We outline a few key findings on how the project has evolved from a response to a student challenge into a multicountry clinical trial project, shifting established community health paradigms.

Mobile as a lens for paradigm shifts and disruptive innovation

Exploring a paradigm shift taught our group to analyze the problem with a new lens. The lens can be technological, systemic, or a combination of the two. The resulting view may undermine established agendas among players.

At the inception of Adhere.IO, the challenge of patient noncompliance was brought forth by a group of public health experts who had been heavily invested in DOTS, the current standard of care. Our response was perceived as radical since it could bypass the community healthcare worker altogether. We were proud of our technology, our impression of their reaction to it was that it represented a threat to their establishment. Traditional stakeholders seemed to label the approach as heretic in private, and based on responses to the press and our own introductions, amateurish. Had we followed their advice, the project would have been very different today. We heard reasonable suggestions for undermining the idea:

- 'You don't have to go through the trouble of giving them a test, just give them food.'
- 'The problem is that community health care workers don't get paid enough. Instead of spending the money on a test, just pay them more.'

We had the luxury of employing a new lens toward the problem because we were not beholden to any stakeholders:

- **No one in the team was being funded to develop the project**. While funding was nonexistent with the exception of a few hundred dollars from the MIT to test out some key concepts, we were completely autonomous.
- **There were no jobs at stake**. All participants either had a day job or were full-time students. This was a completely separate activity with very little overlap, and no shared oversight. This provided a truly free space to explore new approaches. In the long-term, this would later prove to be one of the most difficult aspects of maintaining a healthy continuity of the project.
- It was **not part of a tenure track research agenda**. No one held an academic position at the time of inception. Adhere.IO is interesting from a systems integration and public health perspective. However, the very nature of its simplicity makes it a poor candidate for an engineering or basic science publication on which to base a tenure agenda. The chemistry was known and established in 1972 (Ellard, Gammon and Wallace, 1972). Lateral

flow technology has been around for decades. SMS reminder and healthy behavior messaging systems had already been widely used. In academia, all the above are translated into 'it's already been published'. Had we followed that agenda, the project may have never taken off the ground.

- We had the **benefit of being outsiders** who could look at the problem with a **fresh perspective.** None of us had a public health background. We were designers who had no idea which aspects of the project might run into 'sacred cows' and which questions were naive. Being an outsider allowed us to explore what might be a familiar territory to others.
- **Extensions and expansion of DOTS (the current standard of care) were not part of our metrics for success**. Looking back at the inception of the project, we suspect that some of the promoters of the challenge might have been looking at a method to augment or accelerate the current approaches to tuberculosis compliance it the field. In the end, we took note of those approaches, and became particularly impressed by the high rates of absenteeism presented by Banerjee and Duflo (Banerjee *et al.*, 2006). Our approach shifted the locus of power from the community healthcare worker to the patient.

The structure of the disruption

Previous remote approaches at dealing with lack of adherence have used various methods including reminder systems, incentives, supervisor incentives, and verification. To date, there is no widespread system that combines verification and incentives.

Table 12.1 Conventional approaches to adherence persuasion

	DOTS	**DOTS Incentives**	**xHale**	**Proteus Helium**	**Health Honors**
Reminder					X
Patient incentives					X
Supervisor incentives		X			
Verification			X	X	
Healthcare Professional centric	X				
Patient centric			X	X	X

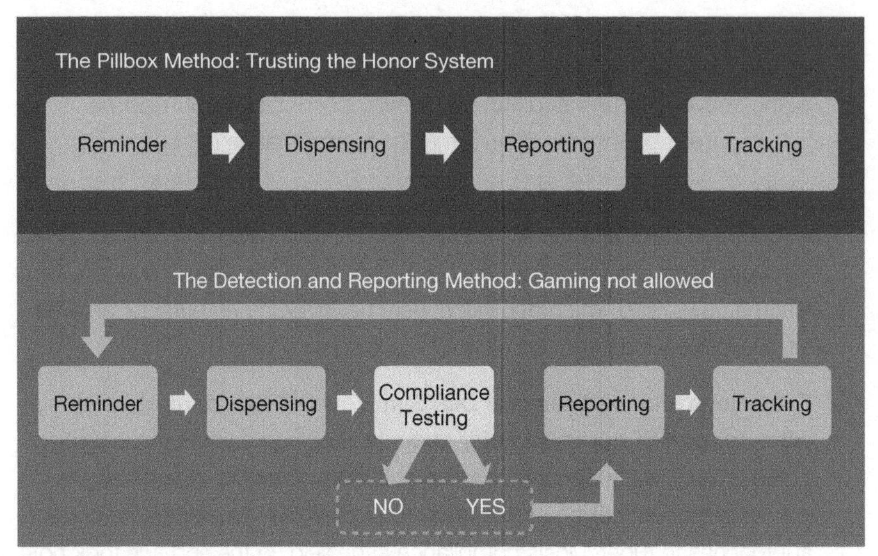

Figure 12.3 Detection and Reporting Method

Many approaches focused on empowering the healthcare worker instead of the patient. This resulted in misdirected incentives, healthcare-centric verification diagnostics, and a declining relationship between the healthcare worker and the patient: less caretaker, more supervisor. Our design for the Adhere.IO ecosystem aims to create a system in which the supervisory role and the caretaker role are decoupled, as shown in Figure 12.1. In order to do that, the patient has to gain a relationship with a third party – the incentive mechanism – that serves as a proxy for supervision and monitoring.

The mobile as a reader

Adhere.IO is part of a growing group of mHealth technologies coupling the communications power of a phone with onboard diagnostics. These are technologies that strive to be independent of a system. We have noted an overwhelming number of mHealth approaches that focus on novel transmission of patient data packets. This approach assumes that we have obtained the right information in the first place. There is space for more innovation in the field for creating these types of hardware apps. Since Adhere.IO's invention, the field of hardware apps on mobiles has grown. In 2009 and 2010, a number of significant innovations in pairing vital signs with mobiles emerged such as ThinkLabs stethoscopes. In 2011, we saw a surge in technologies aimed at pairing wet lab sensors with mobile phones such as the ESTI2 research consortium that develops mobile phone STD tests (Sutter, 2010). Solutions like Adhere.IO strive to take advantage of the phone's ability to do more than serve as a portable database. This creates additional opportunities to interact with a patient's health status, opening gateways for positive behavior change.

Cross-functional team formation

The XoutTB project assembled a team that focused on creating a biosensor-driven system coupled to a telecommunications platform. It required a multidisciplinary team that included chemistry, mechanical engineering, policy, economics, and clinical experience. Beyond creating diversity within the group, we forced cross-functional tasks to avoid attacking the problem conventionally. In fact, we did not have an IT person at the inception of the project.

We applied a Solution Architecture (Gomez-Marquez, 2010) approach to tackling a problem in which we had limited expertise and limited funds. In this way, we sought out help as needed.

Solution architectures

Designing projects for the developing world can attract many forms of assistance both in-kind resources and subject matter expertise (SME). The latter is critical at every stage of a project. It can be helpful to understand the types of expertise you will need to seek and bring together to realize your design. This involves grouping technologies and ideas. It also involves assembling individuals who may be part of your team and other may be participating as mentors.

The mobile as a walkie-talkie

By placing much of the innovation on the sensor, we ended up with a system in which reception of the coded message by the patient can be done in a number of ways, not just a mobile phone. By focusing on the intricacies of the other aspects of the solution, we refused to be tied down to many IT-laden challenges and prevalent discussion points such as debates about open sourced code, data storage mechanisms, SMS versus Data, cloud-based apps versus in-phone software.

During our period of system development, we were able to focus on aspects of chemistry, mechanical engineering, and behavioral economics that would ultimately tie-in to a telecommunications system. This led to telecommunications neutrality. Our aim was to create a messaging and incentive system in which the patient could use a number of communications devices, not just mobile phones, to verify their adherence behavior.

It is conceivable that if we had started with a smartphone, a team of software developers, and a mandate to create something specifically for mobile health, we may have invented a complex piece of hardware and software with rigorous smartphone requirements. Allowing the team to treat the phone system as a walkie-talkie directed the flow of ideas toward the initial sensing and behavior reward scheme.

Bottom-up innovation leads to a change in the incentive scheme

In August 2007, our team arrived in Nicaragua for our first engineering field trial to test the manufacturability of our system. One of the first changes in system design came from Ezequiel Provedor, head of CARE's health division: Use cell-minutes as a reward instead of microfinance credits. That decision shifted our 'telecommunications neutrality' to a definitive bias toward mobile phones. It was a decision based on the incentive system as opposed to the choice of communications technology. The decision created a mobile-centric evolution to the process. At the same time, it swept the project up in the popularity and promise of mobile health. One of our fundamental aims is to separate the hype around mobile technologies for health from the core innovations that create behavior changing technologies.

Surviving the double valley of death for emerging technologies for global health

Appropriate technologies for health can often leave researchers in a quandary: technologies must be simple and affordable, but often simplicity leads the research agenda to be considered less-than-cutting edge for traditional grants and academic funding mechanisms. Our lab describes this as the 'Double Valley of Death'. In medical device commercialization, the Valley of Death is recognized as that period that a technology has to survive in between academic research funding and pre-revenue commercialization activities. In global health, an often overlooked Valley of Death is the period beyond early stage seed funding and mid-stage research where the uncertainty of an idea is still as high as its promise. Adhere.IO has been a classic case of a technology going through both Valleys. The project received an early stage award of less than US $10,000 to develop a refined prototype that included field testing. Additional funds from private donors doubled that amount to a manageable budget for materials and incidentals, but not equipment. After creating reputable bench prototypes, a small US $50,000 NIH Award allowed the project to continue development, and in 2009 a major award for a clinical trial in Pakistan was awarded. The award was later revised to pay for evaluation costs but not for implementation costs. In practice this meant we could pay to evaluate the technology, but we could not pay to actually develop it. This scenario occurs far too often in global health technology research. As more funds are placed in 'mezzanine level' awards instead of early stage awards, promising technologies may simply be abandoned for more sustainable projects. To counteract this trend, we embraced several tactics:

Vintage technologies. Instead of reinventing the chemistry, we scoured proven assays that had worked before and focused on re-contextualizing the solution with today's available technologies – such as mobile phone and paper microfluidics.

Lean prototype fabrication strategies. Our laboratory has specialized in the creation of affordable prototyping methods for a variety of biomedical and diagnostic devices. For instance, early in the project we recognized that instead of expensive filter paper sold by specialty chemical suppliers, we could use generic coffee filters as a substrate.

Trickle-Up Applications. Adhere.IO began as XoutTB, a diagnostic platform intended for tuberculosis adherence. After failing to get early stage funding interest from parties in global health, we took our platform that was already as simple as an interactive diagnostic could get, and applied it toward domestic uses. In the Unites States, nonadherence costs the healthcare system approximately US $290 billion a year in follow-up costs, according to the New England Health Care Institute. The promise of a technology that is simple, affordable, and universally compatible with most telecommunications systems is now very attractive to domestic markets – without losing its soul and intention to help patients in the poorest of countries who are trying to get well from diseases that just need them to change their behavior to stay healthy.

References

Ainslie, G. and Monterosso, J. (2002), 'Hyperbolic Discounting Lets Empathy Be a Motivated Process', *Behavioral and Brain Sciences* 25: 20–1.

Banerjee, A. and Duflo, E. (2006), 'Addressing Absence', *Journal of Economic Perspectives* 20(1): 117–32.

Centers for Disease Control and Prevention (2009), Questions and Answers About TB. Atlanta, Centers for Disease Control and Prevention.

Chaudhury, N., Hammer, J., Kremer, M., Muralidharan, K. and Rogers, F.H. (2006), 'Missing in Action: Teacher and Health Worker Absence in Developing Countries' *The Journal of Economic Perspectives* 20(1): 91–116.

Ellard, G.A., Gammon, P.T. and Wallace, S.M. (1972), 'The Determination of Isoniazid and Its Metabolites Acetylisoniazid, Monoacetylhydrazine, Diacetylhydrazine, Isonicotinic Acid and Isonicotinylglycine in Serum and Urine', *Biochemical Journal* 126(3): 449–58.

Gomez-Marquez, J.F. (2010), Solution Architecture as a Design Strategy. D-Lab Health, Lecture 3. Cambridge, MA, MIT.

Gomez-Marquez, J.F. and Hanumara, N.C. (2010), MultiBDx: A Multiplexed Behavioral Diagnostic Platform, MIT Case No. 14560. Cambridge, MA, MIT.

Haynes, R., McDonald, H., Garg, A. and Montague, P. (2002), 'Interventions for Helping Patients to Follow Prescriptions for Medications', *The Cochrane Database of Systematic Reviews*(2).
Moulding, T.S. (2007), 'Viewpoint: Adapting to New International Tuberculosis Treatment Standards with Medication Monitors and DOT Given Selectively', *Tropical medicine and international health* 12(11): 1302–8.
Sutter, J.D. (2010, 9 November), 'Mobile Phones May Diagnose STDs', *CNN.com*, http://www.cnn.com/2010/TECH/innovation/11/09/diseases.mobile.phone/index.html [Accessed 21 February 2012].
Wandwalo, E., Robberstad, B. and Morkve, O. (2005), 'Cost and Cost-Effectiveness of Community Based and Health Facility Based Directly Observed Treatment of Tuberculosis in Dar Es Salaam, Tanzania', *Cost Effectiveness and Resource Allocation* 3(6).
Ware, N.C., Idoko, J., Kaaya, S., Biraro, I.A., Wyatt, M.A., Agbaji, O., Chalamilla, G. and Bangsberg, D.R. (2009), 'Explaining Adherence Success in Sub-Saharan Africa: An Ethnographic Study', *PLoS Medicine* 6(1).
WHO (2010), *Global Tuberculosis Control 2009*, Geneva: WHO.

13 Conclusion

Patricia Mechael, mHealth Alliance at the UN Foundation and Earth Institute at Columbia University and Jonathan Donner, Microsoft Research

Introduction

In the introduction to this volume on the *State of Behavior Change Initiatives and How Mobile Phones are Transforming It*, Kwan, Mechael, and Kaonga highlight the growing role of mobile communications technologies in public health interventions. Changing human behaviors and attitudes requires time, considerable effort, and motivation; yet for those implementing programs, both the underlying determinants of behavior and the practices supporting the application of strategic communications theory to change campaigns are often not top-of-mind. A recent review by (Riley, Rivera, Atienza, Nilsen, Allison, and Mermelstein, 2011). of the published clinical outcome studies on mobile behavior change initiatives found that explicit linkages to behavioral change theory were more common among antismoking and weight/diet interventions than among treatment adherence and disease management interventions. Indeed, of twenty studies on mobile disease management interventions (in diabetes, asthma, and hypertension), Riley *et al.* found only one with a specific link to behavior change theory. This gap between theory and practice came up repeatedly in the conversations we had with workshop participants in the London sessions, and in the chapters of this volume that grew out of those discussions.

Mobile technologies are unlocking a new mechanism for promoting behavior change. Mobile phones are being used for every stage of disease – from health knowledge and promotion to disease prevention, diagnosis, and treatment, including appointment reminders and medication compliance. Although mobile phones have been the focus of considerable public health research in developed countries (Fogg and Eckles, 2007; Fogg and Adler, 2009), the strengths and limitations of mobile phones in behavior change campaigns in developing countries are less well-understood. This lack of documentation and sharing was reinforced by the projects and research in this volume. While there is a broad range of mHealth behavior change initiatives in low- and middle-income countries from gaming for HIV/AIDS awareness to self-management of diabetes to video support for frontline health workers, there is limited research to evaluate their impact. This edited book provides a snapshot of mobile-mediated behavior change projects emphasizing health promotion and disease prevention as well as disease management, treatment compliance, and appointment reminders and explores the theoretical frameworks that underpin them in a way that examines what 'mobile' brings to the behavior change world and what more there is to understand. This conclusion chapter provides a review and reflection on the projects and research described in the book as well as some insights into where we might want to go from here.

Moving beyond the pilots and hype toward systematic integration of mHealth

Over the last decade, the mobile technology landscape has changed dramatically across the developing world. Mobile phones are enabling higher levels of human capacity and productivity in a range of 'development' domains, from agriculture and education to governance and health (Donner, 2008; Aker, 2010). One theme that emerged from the discussions is how during this initial boom in mobile use, early innovators had been working across a wide set of national contexts and organizational settings, but with little initial awareness of other contemporary efforts. Through the lens of over ten years of mHealth experience in using mobile for HIV and AIDS prevention, care, and support, Peter Benjamin from Cell-Life in South Africa explored the need for communication and how it is this need that has driven the uptake of mobile phones beyond what anyone could have anticipated. For example, van Beijma and Hoefman were quick to recognize the potential to communicate health information to people in low-resource settings via a mobile phone. By 2007, they had proposed and designed a solution implemented by Text to Change (TTC), using short message service (SMS) as an easy, cost-effective and interactive way to communicate information, collect data, and create awareness on health issues, including HIV and AIDS, family planning, and malaria. In the meantime, thousands of miles to the west, Ilta Lange applied a thirty-plus year career in health service delivery and worked in tele-health in Chile to the strategic integration of mobile telephony for diabetes management.

How quickly things change: these pockets of initial innovations and experimentations have been replaced with a global web of interconnected initiatives. Full of workshops, conferences, startups, and RFPs, the mHealth community is burgeoning, so much so that there is the risk of an unhealthy 'hype cycle' surrounding mHealth that needs to be tempered with research, methodical approaches, and the sharing of real stories of success and failure (Fenn and Raskino, 2008). Mobile technologies are only as good as the systems and the programs that they support. With the onslaught of rapid mass communication and mass interaction, almost anyone anywhere can communicate with nearly anyone else, immediately and for a relatively low cost.

Cell-Life has spent nearly ten years developing, testing, and implementing health applications through basic phones and increasingly moving toward the creation of 'smart apps for dumb phones'. These health applications range from basic lifestyle services through general health information to condition-specific services – where much of their work began in the use of mobiles for HIV and AIDS, health administration, to medical consultations and counseling. Modestly, Benjamin comments that they have just started to learn how to use this new technology, where mobile technology provides an opportunity to increase equity in the provision of quality health services. They are now working with the government of South Africa to advise on and develop strategies for more effective integration of mobile technology at a national scale.

Like many countries, Chile is experiencing a dramatic increase in rates of diabetes as well as of diabetes risk factors, such as obesity and a sedentary lifestyle. The government of Chile has committed itself to providing primary care services to the entire population at need – requiring more innovative approaches to service delivery. This led to Lange's early work in tele-health and more recent foray into mHealth. When her work began, the project did not consider mobiles to provide tele-self-management support to patients with Type 2 diabetes, as the cost of communication was three times higher than calling fixed phones. This decision changed very rapidly, as they encountered the continuous interruption of telephone traffic because copper landlines were stolen, which obliged the project to contact patients through their cellphones. Mobile phone contacts, although more expensive, were more convenient because the program could contact patients at the first instance at home, at work or in other places outside their home. In the long run, the process demanded less professional time, which is scarce and of high cost.

As illustrated by Benjamin, we are just learning how to find effective and proven ways to turn these electronic-connected devices in the pockets of billions of youths and adults into means of accessing a range of health and medical services and sources of information that could transform health systems. Different from other forms of telemedicine or electronic health (eHealth), mHealth can address aspects of healthcare beyond the curative. Lange learned through her work in tele-health that mobile phones have become part and parcel of daily life; such as, mobile tools can be used to address chronic illness as well as build health awareness, enhance preventative healthcare, and support well-being and overall wellness as highlighted by Benjamin. This is a much wider agenda for technology in healthcare than ICT and medicine usually cover. However, while cellphones provide a means of reaching a very large number of people, it must be remembered that there are a significant number of people who do not have access to this technology.

Van Beijma and Hoefman take this a step further and provide some concrete recommendations for how to better ground mHealth as it evolves beyond pilots and hype into more systematic integration within health systems. Governments and organizations enthusiastic to implement mHealth should ask themselves: *What problem is mobile going to solve for us? And what has already been done by other organizations?* It cannot just focus on adding an mHealth component to an existing program or campaign; but needs to be fully integrated into the health system and/or program from conception with both scale and sustainability in mind. The future of mobile phone deployment in health is encouraging and growing steadily; however, it cannot be substituted for a weak health system – a good quality and fully equipped health sector is vital to its success. It should be understood that ICTs/mobile phones are just a tool or an enabler to economic development with the biggest opportunities in improving access to quality and timely health information and knowledge. Government should not be mandated to implement mHealth, but act as the overseer, giving support and guidance as much as possible. They should also create an auspicious environment to deploy mHealth by putting policy frameworks and making available essential information and knowledge as often as they can. Approximately four years ago, TTC gave an eye-opening presentation about the potential of using mobile phones in health communication to senior management at Ministry of Health in Uganda and from this it was decided that mHealth be used in their programs.

Development of a strong regulatory framework involving a range of stakeholders with emphasis on end-user involvement is needed and slowly emerging in a number of countries, including Uganda. A national ICT policy is in place and a health sector ICT policy (eHealth) is already operational. The Uganda Ministry of Health is taking steps to coordinate ICT development and has allocated resources to support implementation of its ICT strategy. Nationwide deployment of an mHealth application program could only be successful with the inclusion of government having a dedicated budget. MHealth applications have the potential to improve and strengthen the current health system if integrated into an existing 'well-functioning' structure. As a compliment to emerging regulatory frameworks and policies, new business models and more effective public-private partnerships are needed to solidify the growth and stability of mHealth for behavior change.

The state of mHealth for behavior change research

In early 2010, Heather Cole-Lewis's article entitled 'Text messaging as a tool for behavior change in disease prevention and management' was published in the peer-reviewed journal, *Epidemiologic Reviews* (Cole-Lewis and Kershaw, 2010).

This systematic review of the peer-reviewed literature on behavior change interventions for disease management and prevention delivered through mobile text messaging identified nine out of twelve studies that were sufficiently powered to detect a difference in the intervention conditions. Of those nine, eight studies suggested that text messaging was a useful tool for behavior change. The utility of text messaging was supported for users of different ages, nationalities, and minority status. Only one of the nine countries represented in this study is considered a developing country. The review recorded characteristics of each intervention and attempted to identify the gaps and issues in the literature as well as the best practices for researchers and practitioners. Issues identified include lack of scientific rigor, little representation of developing countries, and lack of use of behavioral theory.

In order to understand why mHealth interventions have an impact, it is important to conceptualize the mechanisms by which we expect change to happen for each specific aspect of the intervention. Using an overall model of change during the design, implementation, and evaluation stages can both inform how a program is positioned and identify how to approach measuring the outcomes one aims to achieve.

There is an ecosystem of health that already exists; the overlay of mobile phones has only made this ecosystem more fluid and is allowing it to progress rapidly. Each mHealth intervention will take a different approach depending on circumstances and the resources available. As summarized by Cole-Lewis, no one project will answer all the questions on mHealth, but if we are able to build upon theoretical models, lessons learned from other ICT and/or health-related research, develop sound and systematic documentation of methods, and apply rigor in evaluations, we will eventually be able to piece it all together.

Mobile messaging: Methods to the madness

A critical challenge often cited in mHealth programs is how best to approach messaging. What is the optimal tone, frequency, and mode of interaction, and what methods are available for evaluating whether they have generated the desired behaviors? Can what has been done in one environment be effectively adapted for use in another? The work of Caroline Free to leverage messaging for smoking cessation in the United Kingdom, Jessica Osborn for maternal and newborn health in Ghana, and Divya Ramachandran for ASHAs promoting health pregnancies in India explores answers to these questions. The work of Free and Ramachandran highlights critical dimensions of a systematic process as applied to mHealth for behavior change, while the work of Osborn provides some critical lessons learned through doing mHealth messaging.

As illustrated by Free, existing effective behavior change smoking cessation support interventions include group, one-on-one, and telephone counseling. However, many smokers cannot or do not want to use existing services. Motivational messages and behavior change tools used in face-to-face smoking cessation support have been modified for delivery via mobile phones with the content tailored to the age, sex, and ethnic group of the quitter (Rodgers, Corbett, Bramley, Riddell, Wills, Lin, and Jones, 2005; Free, Whittaker, Knight, Abramsky, Rodgers, and Roberts, 2009). In this way, support is delivered wherever the person is located, without them having to attend services and can be interactive, allowing quitters to obtain extra help when needed. Because of the widespread ownership of mobile phones, fully automated smoking cessation support can be delivered to large numbers of people at low cost.

The STOMP (Stop smoking with mobile phones) trial, conducted among 1,700 young smokers (at least sixteen years of age, with a mean age of twenty-five years) throughout New Zealand, assessed the effectiveness of a text message-based smoking cessation intervention (Rodgers *et al.*, 2005). It showed considerable promise, with over a twofold increase in self-reported quit rates at six weeks (28 per cent versus 13 per cent, relative risk 2.2, a 95 per cent confidence interval of 1.79 to 2.70, p value of less than 0.0001). The results were consistent and separately significant across all major subgroups including those defined by age, sex, ethnicity, income level, and geographical location. The txt2stop intervention in the United Kingdom was modified and developed from the STOMP intervention and was evaluated in a randomized controlled trial with 5,800 participants (Free, Cairns, Whittaker, and Edwards, 2008; Free *et al.*, 2009), perhaps the largest study of its kind.

Ramachandran used ethnographic research, iterative design, and experimentation with a range of audio-visual aids to help ASHAs communicate with their pregnant clients during house visits and counseling sessions in the poorest state in India, Orissa, which struggles to achieve targeted health outcomes for women and children. The final version of the videos followed a dialogue-based structure, drawing from theories of persuasion, influence, and rhetoric. These videos directly addressed the prevalent myths and barriers that hindered the acceptance and utilization of information and services that ASHAs provided. The videos followed a scripted dialogue, with built-in pauses and questions which ASHAs quickly learned to follow and emulate that led to a significant increase in the ASHAs' ability to provide effective and high-quality counseling, and considerable engagement from clients and their family members.

Through a focus on persuasion during the iterative design process, Ramachandran developed a change model that was pieced together and adapted according to qualitative interviews, lessons from local stakeholders, and iterative field-testing. Six guiding principles for designers of persuasive messages emerged: (1) focus the message on action items, not on broad topics of information, (2) address local myths and barriers, and provide convincing corrections and solutions, respectively, (3) create opportunities for structured, persuasive dialogue between humans, keeping in mind that persuasion is a largely social phenomenon in rural communities, (4) include reminders about the positive rewards for changing behavior, paying close attention to local values, (5) capture the most persuasive local language and prosody style, even if it is counterintuitive, and (6) do not assume reactions are honest – persuasion takes time.

Similar to other authors in this volume, Ramachandran studied a number of different theoretical frameworks, but found that no single one perfectly fitted in the context in which she was working. What she calls a mosaic model emerged through a mix of theory, practice, and intuition is necessary to accommodate factors that can influence the persuasive power of any interaction whether it is human-to-human or human-to-machine.

With a similar focus on pregnant women and their children, the Mobile Technology for Community Health (MOTECH) Initiative as described by Osborn uses two interrelated mobile phone applications to increase the quantity and quality of antenatal and neonatal care in rural Ghana with a specific goal of improving health outcomes for mothers and their newborns. Access to basic health information in rural areas of Ghana is limited, resulting in lack of knowledge about maternal and child health, low uptake of health services, and adherence to often-damaging local myths and cultural practices, contributing to high maternal and child morbidity and mortality. The 'Mobile Midwife' application enables pregnant women and their families to receive SMS or pre-recorded voice messages on personal mobile phones that provide time-specific information about their pregnancy each week. Information is provided in the client's local language and is localized to address issues faced in various regions of the country. The messages continue through the first year of life of the newborn and reinforce well-child care practices and vaccination schedules. The 'Nurse Application' enables Community Health Nurses to electronically record care given to patients and identify women and newborns in their area that are due for care. MOTECH has linked its two mobile applications so that if a patient has missed treatment that is part of the defined care schedule, the Mobile Midwife service sends an appointment reminder to the patient and nurse.

Existing guidance for the development and evaluation of complex interventions suggests that key elements of the process include development, feasibility and piloting, evaluation, and implementation phases (Craig, Dieppe, Macintyre, Michie, Nazareth, and Petticrew, 2008). Unlike many other mHealth projects and evaluations (as illustrated by Cole-Lewis and Riley (Cole-Lewis and Kershaw, 2010; Riley *et al.*, 2011)), the work of Free *et al.* was approached systematically beginning with theory, the existing evidence base and the existing STOMP program to generate text messages which were evaluated and modified using feedback from smoking cessation counselors and potential participants in focus groups. The messages were subsequently tested in a pilot trial. Feasibility of the trial process (recruitment, follow up) and delivery of the intervention were assessed in a pilot trial. Findings from the process evaluation for the pilot trial were used to further develop the intervention. The intervention was subsequently evaluated in a main trial. The movement between development, piloting, and evaluation phases provided necessary and critical insights to finalize the txt2stop intervention evaluated in the main trial. Plans for implementation have been initiated. A similar methodology is highly recommended for the development of other texting messaging interventions.

Similar to the work of Free, Osborn identifies common themes to designing applications for specific types of users – those who are consumers of health information and services – in this case pregnant women and their families and those working to provide health services in organizational settings. When designing for consumers, the recognized lack of information drives demand for service which is seen as something with potential for personal benefit (being more informed, having better health). In order to deliver messages to this population, it is critical to use a technology and functionality familiar to the user to enable uptake. In this case, the program expended its plan to use SMS only to provide the same content by voice. The intervention works because it slots into the everyday routines of the user. One debate that often arises in mHealth is whether or not to distribute mobile phones as part of the intervention. There is no apparent business model that makes the provision of mobile phones a viable option, forcing dependency on common channels – voice and SMS. The information service has credibility through its association with respected partners, such as the Ghana Health Service, whom people trust to provide accurate information and is delivered as a standalone effort but one that complements other parallel behavior change initiatives and provides a link to appropriate services.

In the case of delivering mHealth services to health workers, a critical lesson is to begin with a demand for the proposed service that comes from within the organization. This does not always translate into recognition of the need for a technology intervention by individuals within the system, who may not see the personal benefit or gain personal satisfaction from doing a thorough job. This presents a challenge to uptake and compliance, and can limit the success of efforts to encourage that. Related to this is the allowance of the need for changes to existing workflows, which makes it more difficult to integrate the service into the routines of health workers than for their clients. In relation to nurses, the total cost of ownership is reduced by providing phones, enabling the use of data and more sophisticated apps. Credibility has been gained only through demonstrating the Ghana Health Service ownership of the intervention, and ensuring that it is situated in an existing ecosystem. For instance, phones cannot have an impact unless they are implemented alongside efforts to improve service delivery and the appropriate levels of training are provided.

Innovations to inform the next phase of mHealthy behavior change

The works of Sultan and Moran, Quraishi and Quraishi, and Gomez-Marquez illustrate many of the new possibilities emerging within mHealth for behavior change in developing countries, including the use of smartphone applications for self-management of chronic illness in the Caribbean; gaming for health; and treatment compliance for TB treatment through the use of at home mobile phone supported urinalysis. These initiatives represent the engagement of the technology field in helping to introduce innovation within the health sector, raising some recommendations for how to better engage with the health sector and end-users as part of the design process.

Mohan and Sultan's MediNet Project began in 2007 as a response to a Microsoft External Research Request for Proposals, whose theme was 'Cell phone as a Platform for Health Care'. The main objective of the project was to develop a Caribbean-wide healthcare management system that would pool the heathcare resources of the Caribbean Islands, including a mobile phone-based remote patient monitoring and self-management system for chronic illnesses such as diabetes and cardiovascular disease. Sultan and Mohan's main advice to software programmers entering this domain: that while the health sector provides enormous potential and scope for the development of software technology, the intended users of the software must always be considered in the development process and user interfaces should be designed as simply as possible. Systems should concentrate on the value that intended users will gain from using the system rather than having impressive hard-to-use features which are seldom used. It is also important to become familiar with healthcare standards and government regulations and understand the implications they have on the software being developed. A broad range of software development skills are required depending on the target delivery platform and programmers need to develop expertise in many of them. Engaging with a multidisciplinary team is very important, given the many facets of software development associated with a healthcare system and the different stakeholders involved.

For Quraishi and Quraishi, Freedom HIV/AIDS began as a mobile games-based social venture designed to create information and awareness and behavior change among youths on issues related to sexual interaction, myths, and misconceptions surrounding the disease, combating discrimination, and testing and treatment behaviors. With HIV and AIDS, many behavioral practices exist due to lack of information, social-economic conditions, and personal attitudes among the youths contributing to nonconforming behaviors to the facts. Before launching the initiative, a systematic study of types of games popular with the youths, the level of information on the subject and basic general risk behavior trends among the youth was conducted. As the initiative was designed to leverage mobile networks and their reach, games were developed to address these issues based on the highest common factors (HCF) approach as against lowest common multiples to cover a large audience group (gamers both casual and serious).

The initiative was launched on December 1, 2005, on the World AIDS Day, as a gift to Indian youths. Highlighting the benefits of public–private partnerships, ZMQ partnered with the state of Delhi, the Delhi State AIDS Control Society, and Reliance Infocomm – one of the largest mobile operators in India. Over the period, many more partners from all sectors joined the initiative to make it a success. Later, the initiative was scaled to different parts of Africa under the Africa Reach program of ZMQ to address other communicable diseases such as tuberculosis and malaria and other lifestyle diseases such as diabetes, and cancer. While overall, gaming is proving to be a popular approach to create effective learning outcomes, there is much to learn about behavior change pathways, that it is stimulating.

Adhere.IO is a technology invented at the MIT that introduces a new class of medical devices called behavioral diagnostics. Behavioral diagnostics combine emerging trends in applied behavioral economics and diagnostic design at the micro-scale wrapped in a telemedical application. Adhere.IO's application of behavioral diagnostics is a home-based test aimed at improving poor adherence of complex drug regimens such as HIV and tuberculosis. Originally developed with resource-constrained regions (such as Nicaragua) in mind, Adhere.IO's initial deployments may end up in the US domestic market.

Looking across these initiatives, it is already evident that 'behavior change' does not begin and end with reminders, information; nor must it rely on ubiquitous text messaging and USSD channels to be relevant in emerging markets. In the developed world, land of smartphones and copious bandwidth, the mHealth community is witnessing an explosion of innovation in different platforms and programs, coupled with a deeper – albeit still not universal – understanding of the psychological process for behavioral support (from peer groups to behavioral reinforcement) (Fogg and Adler, 2007; Fogg and Eckles, 2009; Riley *et al.*, 2011). The work of Adhere.IO, ZMQ, and MediNet illustrate how similar processes can take root in resource-constrained communities, as well. Data-enabled feature phones and smartphones are becoming more affordable, putting them reach of many more (but still not all) users throughout the developing world.

But this explosion in capabilities presents as great a challenge as it does an opportunity; just because technical functionalities are increasing, there is no guarantee that they will be accompanied by the links to behavioral theory and best practice necessary to get the most out of them; if anything, the new technologies may obscure how many more elements of psychology, sociology, and economics are at play in the design of multimedia, interactive, wireless digital behavior change initiatives. As voice, image, and video join the humble SMS, and as interactivity, presence, and context-aware computation replace one-way 'message blasting', the set of options and genres is expanding. Riley *et al.* described the evolving challenge this way: 'The development of time-intensive, interactive, and adaptive health behavior interventions via mobile technologies demands more intra-individual dynamic regulatory processes than represented in our current health behavior theories' (Riley *et al.*, 2011). Continued knowledge sharing, theoretical linkage and evaluation, critical reflection, and exchange will help the next wave of mHealth innovators deploy and scale more quickly and to great effect.

Conclusion

mHealth for behavior change innovations has become a new buzz word in the public health field throughout the world. In low- and middle-income countries, efforts to leverage mobile phones to provide health information, improve knowledge, and engage individuals in healthier behaviors that generate improved health outcomes are rapidly growing along with more and better research to enhance the impact it is having. This volume is a timely attempt to glean wisdom and learning from early pioneers to better inform decisions related to funding, designing, implementing, and evaluating such programs, and to minimize the reinvention of the wheel and learning the hard way. While it was challenging for many of the practitioners represented in this book to step back and reflect on their experiences, their contributions throughout the process have been tremendous. It is their voices and on-the-ground insights that will help us all become more thoughtful in our approaches to this work and ultimately generate programs that are more fully integrated in a meaningful way into the everyday lives of those who *are* well to *stay* well, and those who fall ill to better manage their health.

References

Aker, J. (2010), 'Information from Markets near and Far: Mobile Phones and Agricultural Markets in Niger', *American Economic Journal: Applied Economics* 2(3): 46–59.

Cole-Lewis, H. and Kershaw, T. (2010), 'Text Messaging as a Tool for Behavior Change in Disease Prevention and Management', *Epidemiologic Reviews* 32(1): 56–69.

Craig, P., Dieppe, P., Macintyre, S., Michie, S., Nazareth, I., Petticrew, M. and Guidance, M.R.C. (2008), 'Developing and Evaluating Complex Interventions: The New Medical Research Council Guidance', *BMJ* 337: a1655.

Donner, J. (2008), 'Research Approaches to Mobile Use in the Developing World: A Review of the Literature', *The Information Society* 24(3): 140–59.

Fenn, J. and Raskino, M. (2008), *Mastering the Hype Cycle: How to Choose the Right Innovation at the Right Time*, Boston: Harvard Business School Publishing.

Fogg, B. and Adler, R. (2009), *Texting 4 Health: A Simple, Powerful Way to Change Lives*, Stanford: Captology Media.

Fogg, B. and Eckles, D. (2007), *Mobile Persuasion: 20 Perspectives of the Future of Behavior Change*, Stanford: Captology Media.

Free, C., Cairns, J., Whittaker, R. and Edwards, P. (2008), 'Txt2stop: A Randomised Trial of Cell-Phone Text-Messaging to Support Cessation in the UK', *The Lancet* Protocol Reviews.

Free, C., Whittaker, R., Knight, R., Abramsky, T., Rodgers, A. and Roberts, I. (2009), 'Txt2stop: A Pilot Randomised Controlled Trial of Mobile Phone-Based Smoking Cessation Support', *Tobacco Control* 18(2): 88–91.

Riley, W., Rivera, D., Atienza, A., Nilsen, W., Allison, S. and Mermelstein, R. (2011), 'Health Behavior Models in the Age of Mobile Interventions: Are Our Theories up to the Task?', *Translational Behavioral Medicine* 1(1): 53–71.

Rodgers, A., Corbett, T., Bramley, D., Riddell, T., Wills, M., Lin, R. and Jones, M. (2005), 'Do U Smoke after Txt? Results of a Randomised Trial of Smoking Cessation Using Mobile Phone Text Messaging', *Tobacco Control* 14(4): 255–61.

Index